BEREAVEMENT –
A GUIDE FOR NURSES

BEREAVEMENT –
A GUIDE FOR NURSES

Jenny Penson, MA, (Ed), SRN, HVCert, Cert Ed, RNT
Lecturer at the Dorset Institute of Higher Education,
and former Macmillan Nurse

Harper & Row, Publishers
London

Philadelphia
New York
St. Louis
Sydney

San Francisco
London
Singapore
Tokyo

First published 1990

Harper & Row Ltd
Middlesex House
34–42 Cleveland Street
London W1P 5FB

British Library Cataloguing in Publication Data
Penson, Jenny
  Bereavement — a guide for nurses. (Lippincott nursing
  series).
  1. Bereaved persons. Counselling
  I. Bereavement — a guide for nurses
  362.8

  ISBN 0-06-318440-0

Typeset by Burns & Smith Ltd., Derby
Printed in Great Britain at the Alden Press, Oxford

For Jonathon

Contents

Introduction   ix
Acknowledgements   xiii

1. Bereavement – What Is It?   1
2. Culture, Customs and Rituals   16
3. Family Needs: Before the Death of the Patient   27
4. Family Needs: At the Time of the Patient's Death   45
5. Prolonged or Complicated Mourning   61
6. At Risk Groups: Death at the Beginning of Life – Death
   and Children   73
7. At Risk Groups: Death in Adulthood   92
8. Family Needs after the Death   110
9. What Can We Do to Help?: Care in the Community   118
10. How Can We Help? – The Skills of Communication   136
11. The Way Forward: Selection, Support and Education
    for Nurses   154

Appendices: Useful Addresses   166
             Further Reading   169

Index   171

Introduction

They say one must keep your standards and your values alive. But how can I, when I only kept them for you?

Everything was for you.

I loved life because you made it so perfect, and now there is no-one left to make jokes with, or to talk about Racine and Molière, and talk about plans and work and people.

I dreamt of you again last night. And when I woke up it was as if you had died afresh.

Every day I find it harder to bear.

For what point is there in life now?

I look at our favourites, I try and read them, but without you they give me no pleasure. I only remember the evenings when you read to me aloud and I cry.

I feel as if we had collected all our wheat into a barn to make bread and beer for the rest of our lives and now the barn has burnt down and we stand on a cold winter morning looking out at the charred ruins.

For this little room was the gleanings of our life together.

All our happiness was over this fire and with these books.

With Voltaire blessing us with upraised hand on the wall . . . .

It is impossible to think that I shall never sit with you again and hear you laugh.

That every day for the rest of my life you will be away.

(from Dora Carrington's diaries, dated 12–17 February 1932. Lytton

Strachey died in January 1932. Dora Carrington killed herself in March 1932. Printed with kind permission of the estate of David Garnett, the Sophie Partridge Trust)

This short extract very effectively conveys the anguish and sense of desolation which accompanies the loss of someone much loved. When one reads such descriptions or talks with recently bereaved people, one has to ask if there is anything at all that anyone can do to ease that emotional pain. As nurses, we are trained to alleviate physical pain and to support our patients through psychological pain. We are increasingly becoming involved with patients' relatives, whether we are hospital nurses, meeting them on the wards, in intensive care, accident and emergency departments, or if we are community nurses working in their homes or as midwives and health visitors working with families.

What, if anything, have we to offer them? Is there anything we can do *before* the death of the patient that may help his relatives later? Should we be involved in supporting these people afterwards? If so, what should we be doing? What does this overworked word 'support' really mean? Is the nurse the key person to help the bereaved or are there others who should be involved? Death is a natural and inevitable life event so should bereavement be an issue for nurses to consider at all?

If we do so our overall aim is to attempt to help bereaved people towards adjustment to their loss. Is this too tall an order? How will we, as nurses, cope with the certainty that some people will *never* adjust and will suffer the pain of grief for the rest of their lives?

These are some of the issues which I intend to address in this book. It was conceived in response to the concern expressed by so many nurses, working in both hospital and community, district nurses and health visitors, specialist Macmillan and hospice nurses, midwives and community psychiatric nurses whom I have met at the large number of conferences and study days in which I have participated over the last seven years, both in England and abroad.

It is written with the hope that increased knowledge and reflection will enable nurses to meet these needs and to feel comfortable about this within themselves. It may also be seen as an educational exercise. If so, I intend it to be considered in the light of the true meaning of that word, 'education', which is derived from the Latin *educare* – to bring out what is already there.

Writing a book about bereavement is to write a book about life; if there was no life there would be no bereavement. So how can we help bereaved people to return to life, to live with their loss? How should we, as nurses, respond? How can we support them?

To achieve this:

- We need knowledge of what bereavement is, what is usual, some different perspectives (Chapter 1).
- We need to enhance this knowledge by looking at different customs, cultures and rituals (Chapter 2).
- We need to be able to understand the needs of bereaved people before the death of the patient (where this is possible) (Chapter 3), at the time of death (Chapter 4) and afterwards (Chapter 8).
- We need to be able to recognize signs of prolonged or complicated mourning (Chapter 5).
- We need to be made aware of the special needs of people who appear to be at risk (Chapters 6 and 7).
- We need, where necessary, to be able to give continuity of care *after* the death of the patient (Chapter 8).
- We need to be aware of, and sometimes to offer, many different kinds of help (Chapter 9).
- In order to do this, we need communication and other interpersonal skills (Chapter 10).
- As carers we need support and education ourselves (Chapter 11).

Like most authors of books for nurses, I have been faced with the problem of deciding how to express the gender of both nurses and patients. In spite of the growing number of male nurses and of the increasing percentage of men in senior nurse posts, the majority of nurses are still female. Therefore, I have chosen to refer to all nurses as 'she' and, where gender is not specified, all patients are referred to as 'he'. I hope that male readers of this book will bear with me!

The other dilemma I faced was in deciding how to refer to bereaved people in terms of their relationship to the person who died. In choosing to use words such as 'family' or 'relatives', I do not wish to imply that someone only distantly related or not even related at all to the one who died, has not been bereaved. Terms such as 'key person' or 'significant other' may more accurately describe the one who is most affected by the loss. This person could be a lifelong friend, a caring neighbour, an aunt who happens to be closer to the dying person than her mother, the grandparent who virtually brought the person up, the common-law husband or wife, the homosexual lover, the mistress or lover. For simplicity I have used the words 'family' and 'relatives' to encompass anyone who is deeply affected by a person's bereavement, whether they were related to the person who died, or not.

Acknowledgements

First, I would like to thank the many bereaved people who, by being willing to share their feelings and needs with me, have enabled me to share their experiences with you. I would also like to take this opportunity of acknowledging the support, information, advice and time which many nurses and other colleagues have given me.

I would particularly like to thank Dr Roland Fisher, former Consultant in charge of the Macmillan Unit, Christchurch Hospital, Dorset, now Honorary Consultant Physician to the National Society for Cancer Relief, for his inspiration, interest and practical help. I would also like to thank Miss Olga Craig, medical social worker, whose wisdom borne of experience influenced the attitudes expressed.

I would like to thank Griselda Campbell, Editor, Harper and Row, for her understanding and support.

A big thank you to Angela Spoors, Computer Services Unit, Dorset Institute, who unravelled my muddled writing and helped to create a clear and pleasing presentation.

Not least of all I would like to thank my family who have cheerfully put up with my preoccupations and have coped magnificently with my absences.

1. Bereavement – What Is It?

To fear death, gentlemen, is nothing other than to think oneself wise when one is not, for it is to think one knows what one does not know. No man knows whether death may not turn out to be the greatest of blessings for a human being; and yet people fear it as if they knew for certain that it is the greatest of evils.

Socrates (Greek philosopher, 399–470 BC)

INTRODUCTION

Bereavement is an experience which is likely to happen to all of us at some time in our lives. Already, in your professional life you will have felt sorrow at the death of a patient you have nursed for some time, or the unexpected loss of a patient who was getting better, or the death of someone whose age or situation reminded you of your own. These kinds of deaths will have touched you – but from a distance. If you have experienced bereavement yourself, that is the loss of someone whom you loved, then you will know that it is a devastating event, shattering your confidence in the future and changing your life forever. Every facet of your being and each element of your way of life is inexorably altered for all time. You will never be the same person that you were and you may not want to be. Your attitudes to life and your priorities may also have been permanently changed.

The word 'bereavement' means 'to be robbed of something valued'.

I find this a very helpful definition as it indicates that this someone has been wrongfully and forcibly taken away from you. You should not have had to lose them. As they have been unfairly taken away from you it is understandable that the experience of being bereaved is one of strong, overwhelming and sometimes even violent reactions.

The key concept for understanding bereavement is that of loss. Caplan (1964) suggests that the emotions felt after losing someone you love are similar to those felt after other kinds of losses. Any one of you reading this book will have experienced some kind of loss and thinking back to how you felt may help you to empathize with the feelings of bereaved people. You may notice that I do not use the word 'understand' here. I suggest that it is rarely an appropriate word to use even if we too have been bereaved. The grief each person feels is a unique part of them. Therefore no-one else can completely understand another's pain.

DIVORCE

Your experience of loss may have been through divorce or separation. Often this involves other losses such as moving away from members of family, friends and a familiar community. Marriage breakdown is a kind of death. Divorce evokes as intense emotions as bereavement; feelings of anger may be particularly strong and there is a sense of being abandoned by someone who deliberately chose to leave. Some divorced people say they wish that their partner had died instead of having to live with constant disagreements, jealousy and a sense of failure. Feelings of stigma (usually associated with the older generation) and self-blame may last for the person's lifetime.

Resentment and regret may colour the children's lives also. They may feel the need to support the parent with whom they live and may direct all their angry feelings at the other one. Sometimes these targets are reversed, the parent they live with receiving all the difficult emotions and the other one being supported, perhaps even idolized. Thus the conflicts of the marriage may continue after it has officially 'died'.

Many of you may also be able to recall your feelings at the death of a much-loved pet. Here too the loss is of a part of your life as well as of the animal itself. 'It marked the end of my childhood,' said a colleague, describing the death of her dog. You may remember feelings of loss when you left home for the first time and perhaps moved into the nurses' home when you began your training. Therefore we may mourn the loss of what we once had, what we once were, what we hoped might be.

It has also been suggested that even the loss of a precious object can provoke reactions of grief; it is not the object itself but what it represents for that individual, that causes the grief. This may be illustrated by a patient I nursed in the gynaecological ward who was admitted for surgery in a very anxious state. She had lost her engagement ring just before she left home. This became the focus for her fear throughout the time she was in hospital because it symbolized her husband's love and care.

As nurses, our contact with the bereaved is usually with the 'next of kin', but we have to bear in mind that many other people may be affected by the death of the patient. Think for a moment about who would be affected if you died. Your husband or boyfriend and parents may be obvious examples, but what about your best friend, your closest colleagues, those immediately senior and junior to you, your grandparents, aunts and uncles, cousins, your nextdoor neighbour, your vicar or priest, teacher or family doctor. If you were ill first, then many people who cared for you during your illness would also be affected in some way.

In our work, it is necessary for us to be aware of the feelings of loss that many of our patients experience as a result of their illness or treatment. Bereavement can be likened to the loss of body image and function that occurs after a colostomy, for example, or a mastectomy. Disease processes often involve loss. One can think of the loss of independence of the patient with multiple sclerosis, the loss of function of the arthritic patient, the loss of choice of lifestyle of the patient with a severe heart attack or the multiple losses of the patient with advanced cancer who has to try to come to terms with the potential loss of life itself.

The loss felt after the amputation of a limb provides a fitting example of this link. When you are bereaved, you have lost a part, and sometimes a very substantial part, of yourself. Everything you shared with that person can never be repeated with anyone else. You have indeed lost part of yourself.

Let us look at three approaches to understanding what happens during bereavement. These are intended as descriptions that may enhance our sensitivity to what is happening, signposts to guide us if and when we are with bereaved people. The proposition that grieving is a predictable, orderly pattern of responses has been made by Parkes (1972), Worden (1984), and Bowlby (1961), who approach grief as if it were a process of recovery from illness.

The best known example of this approach is that of Parkes (1972) who sees the nature of grieving as a process - a rather overworked word in nursing circles! However, what is meant here is that bereavement is made up of a sequence of reactions and this is emphasized by the designation of stages. He describes the bereavement process as being 'the cost of commitment', a very appropriate expression of the idea that life is about balance, often between positive and negative aspects. Therefore, when we open ourselves up to happiness we are inevitably also open to pain. Yet there is another side of this coin as Pincus (1976) points out, 'there is no loss that cannot lead to gain'. Parkes (1972) also said that 'in the flux of life, the individual undergoes many changes, arriving, departing, growing, declining, achieving, failing – every change must involve a loss and a gain'. Thus this balance can be restored.

BEREAVEMENT AS A PROCESS (based on Parkes, 1972)

Phase 1: Shock, numbness and the pain of grieving

For everyone who experiences the death of a loved one, there is first of all a sense of shock and we need to remember that this may be felt even when the death has been long expected. Therefore, the relative may appear either to overreact by feeling faint, crying uncontrollably or clinging to the dead person, or to underreact by appearing very controlled and calm or showing no emotion at all. The latter approach can easily be misconstrued. I can remember one student nurse who felt great hostility towards the husband of a patient she nursed who reacted to her death with coldness and detachment. This initial shock may last for several days, allowing the relative to cope, often very efficiently, with all the necessary practicalities, and to carry them through the ordeal of the funeral.

It is not until this has started to wear off that the bereaved person begins to feel the physical intensity of their loss and only then can they begin the long process of coming to terms with it.

Mind and body are not two separate entities, as we well know, and each influences the other. Grief is felt as a very physical pain and symptoms such as chest tightness, palpitations, shortness of breath, loss of appetite and insomnia are frequent complaints. A restlessness and inability to concentrate may also be felt. Mrs B described this to me as not even being able to sit still long enough to watch 'Coronation Street' (her favourite TV serial which she had followed for years) and feeling as if she was constantly looking for her husband, although she knew that this was 'ridiculous'.

Where the patient was ill for a period before death, the bereaved relative may experience physical symptoms of a similar nature. For example, Miss B, the last remaining member of a large family, nursed her sister at home for several weeks before she died. This sister had carcinoma of the pancreas and suffered intermittent colicky pains and diarrhoea. Miss B complained of these same symptoms throughout the first two years of her bereavement and was eventually fully investigated at the local hospital, but no evidence of disease was found.

The pain of grief is also experienced as a sense of isolation and loneliness. Often this begins with nursing the ill person at home which, in spite of the help that is available in the community, involves a drastic change of lifestyle and the commitment of caring throughout the 24 hours. If the patient is in hospital then life revolves around long daily visits. There is usually a need to take on the obligations and chores normally performed by the patient. The practicalities of daily living, plus the emotional energy directed at the present situation and the changed expectations of the future, tend to separate the bereaved person from others even before the death of the loved one.

Phase 2: Manifestations of fear, guilt, anger and resentment

These strong feelings may override the bereaved person and this is the time when some may be afraid of becoming unstable or mentally ill. It is often a relief for them to be able to express these and to find that they are not, as Lindemann (1944) put it 'uniquely wicked' and also not uncommon.

Fear is felt as insecurity or a longing to escape from reality and it may show itself in anxiety over apparent trivialities, fussiness over small details or in actual panic attacks, which happen when fear and anxiety overwhelm the individual, often in specific situations such as waiting at a bus stop, walking around a supermarket or leaving the house to have coffee with a friend.

The majority of bereaved people seem to experience guilt. If we think of our own relationships we quickly realize that just as we are not perfect no relationship is ideal and that if we looked for reasons to feel guilty we would be likely to find some.

Most bereaved people appear to have the need to express guilt – they may wish they had expressed their feelings more openly or that they had encouraged the loved one to fulfil their ambitions or interests more forcibly. With a long-term illness such as cancer, many express guilt for not interpreting the early signs of the disease as being potentially serious. They often state that they should have insisted their partner saw their doctor much earlier, that they have tended to ignore small early signs of ill-health and may have even encouraged them, for example, to paint the house, or to go on holiday which they did not feel well enough to do.

Guilt may also be felt for stopping mourning. A volunteer bereavement visitor (herself a widow) expressed this well: 'I don't want him to go, and so long as I feel the pain, he will stay alive for me. And when the hurting stops, death becomes final. So many cling to pain. Maybe time, hopefully, will erase that.'

Some may even feel guilty because they blamed the dead person for leaving them. An example that brought this home to me was a one-time prosperous nightclub owner, married with four children. During his illness he became bankrupt and they were forced to move from fairly affluent surroundings to temporary council accommodation in a very poor area. His wife and I were with him when he died at home. Her first words after his death were said with great bitterness, 'How *could* he go and leave me like this?' Later she shared intense feelings of guilt for putting her anger into words at that moment.

Anger may be directed at many different targets. Doctors and, to a lesser extent, nurses may sometimes be blamed and this may not be inappropriate if we remember that our primary function is seen to be to cure the patient. If the patient dies then there has been a failure to cure them, death has not been prevented and has, in a sense, been allowed to happen. It becomes understandable, therefore, that anger directed at the caring professions tends to centre on wards and departments where the relative first begins to realize, or is directly told, that the patient has died or is not going to be cured. The accident and emergency department, the coronary care unit, the surgical ward and radiotherapy unit are all targets for relatives' anger. I am sure you can think of some from your own experience. It points to the need for us, as nurses, to be aware of the negative feelings that may underlie either direct or overt criticism of our colleagues in other wards, departments, or in the community. The relatives' perception of events may well be coloured by the strength of the emotions felt at that time, whether this was when they were told of either the death of the patient or the seriousness of their illness, or the time when they themselves began to realize the likely outcome of that illness.

Patients facing up to chronic or terminal illness are also experiencing feelings of loss. An extreme example of this situation is Mrs M, a patient I visited at home. She was an Austrian lady in her mid 50s, married with a grown-up family, and she had cancer of the breast with metastases. My first visit was one hot summer's day when I sat and roasted in her conservatory while she listed for me all the current targets for her angry feelings. Finally, she leant towards me, eyes blazing, and said 'And do you know what my doctor said to me? He told me I had cancer! What a terrible thing to say to someone when it is not true!' Her general practitioner was a particularly caring doctor with excellent communication skills but Mrs M maintained her anger towards him, and incidentally her extreme denial, throughout the fifteen months of her illness.

Another common target for anger is God. Many bereaved people make such statements as 'He was such a good man', 'She was always helping other people', 'Everyone loved him', 'She was just an innocent child', and these indicate the feeling that God has in some way let that person down, has not kept His side of a bargain. Even those who profess to have a religious faith may go through doubts and anger at this time. Even those who claim to have no religious beliefs at all may also find themselves using God as a target.

Family members and close friends can also find they are on the receiving end of bitter and resentful emotions. The bereaved person may remind them of disputes, disagreements and family feuds, the focus sometimes being the reading of the will. This can be particularly destructive just when the bereaved person most needs the understanding and support of those closest to them. Mr J, who lost his wife after a short illness, directed all his anger at his only daughter, a teenager, reminding her of past real or imagined misbehaviour and confronting her with the belief that she had caused her mother stress which was responsible for her heart attack. This was very destructive for them both and they needed long-term help.

When anger is directed inwards to the bereaved person himself or herself, guilt and fear are felt. Many of us are socialized into not showing our negative emotions to others, so it may be expressed in other ways such as constant irritation and similar symptoms of tension.

Phase 3: Disengagement, apathy and aimlessness

The disengagement from the usual pattern of daily life that often takes place before the death of the loved one can lead to feelings of apathy. Plans are impossible to make, the future seems uncertain or even frightening and the effort required to get through the day seems futile. Bereaved people will often speak of being depressed, but there may be some confusion as to whether they are referring to sadness rather than to a depressed state as these words are often used interchangeably.

Sad feelings are concentrated on the realization of all that can never be, and memories tend to stir up sadness at the beginning. Often we may find, as nurses, that relatives cannot help but dwell on all the sad events that led up to the patient's death, they remember in detail every aspect of the illness and treatment. It may take many months before a bereaved person is able to work through this sufficiently to be able to put it on one side, and only then do they seem able to go further back to happier times (if these did indeed exist); then they can begin to find comfort and pleasure from those memories, even though they may be poignant. By labelling this sadness as depression we may inadvertently encourage the idea that these feelings are abnormal or an illness rather than the sadness that inevitably accompanies the usual bereavement process.

The distress and passivity of this stage contrasts with the strong and sometimes violent feelings of the preceding one.

Phase 4: Gradual hope and a move in new directions

At last, after the negativity of the other three stages, this last one has a positive message. In order to reach this it is necessary to have gone some way towards accepting the reality of the loss. Only then can the bereaved person let go of some of the past and make the first steps towards a new pattern of living. There is a sense of resurrection, of the 'phoenix rising from the ashes', because out of all the sadness and longing eventually comes a new form of life and a realization that what was once a part of you cannot actually be taken from you. It will be part of you forever.

Sometimes this kind of revelation comes quite suddenly to the bereaved person, more often it is a very gradual part of the process. Either way there is for most people some kind of turning point. C. S. Lewis (1961) who mourned the death of his wife, eloquently described this experience: '. . . something quite unexpected has happened. It came this morning early. My heart was lighter than it had been for many weeks . . . suddenly at the very moment when so far I mourned her least, I remembered her best. It was as if the lifting of the sorrow removed a barrier.'

Although we have looked at bereavement in terms of stages we cannot make the assumption that each bereaved person will move neatly from one stage to another. Responses may overlap or merge at times. Sometimes there will be regression to earlier stages. It may be most useful to think in terms of components, some of which will predominate earlier in the process and others later.

An alternative view is based on the work of Worden (1984), who as an American views bereavement positively, implying that the bereaved person is able to influence his experience and that the onus is on the individual to help himself. Like Parkes, he sees grief as an illness. In his view, recovery is achieved via a series of tasks. This is linked with Freud's concept of grief-work.

BEREAVEMENT AS A SERIES OF TASKS

To accept the reality of the loss

It is not until the bereaved person has faced up to the fact that the dead person can never return, in this life at least, that they can begin the task of adjustment. It is suggested that in our society we do not help the accomplishment of this task because, for example, we even avoid referring to the fact that the person has died. We use many euphemisms to avoid the word death such as 'passed over', 'gone across', 'gone to heaven', and we do not encourage the bereaved to talk about what has happened or to show how they are feeling.

To experience pain and grief

This is very painful and it is understandable that the very intensity of these feelings make us want to distract the bereaved person. Gorer (1965) suggests that the expression of grief is stigmatized in our society as being a morbid and unhealthy thing to do. Distraction may work in the short-term but it would appear to be unhelpful long-term as this merely puts off the experience. It is suggested that attempts to short-circuit these feelings rarely work in the long-term and they may lead to deep-seated problems in the future.

To adjust to a new environment

The environment is suddenly strange and new because the deceased person is missing from it. All the roles the deceased person played in it are missing. For example, the newly bereaved mother of young children who has lost her husband has also lost her companion, lover, childminder, accountant, driver and drain-cleaner! It can be salutory to reflect for a moment the number of roles performed in your life by the person closest to you.

Whatever they are, they will include one universal role, that of audience. We all use those closest to us as an audience for our ideas, a sounding board for our plans, hopes and dreams and to reflect back to us the kind of person that we are. Here again we can see that when we lose someone close to us, we lose part of ourselves so that we may no longer know who we are.

To withdraw emotional energy and reinvest it in other relationships

This ties in with Freud's (1957) statement that 'the function of mourning is to detach the survivor's memories and hopes from the dead person'. Freud sees this work as difficult and slow, a painful inner process of letting go. This is considered to be the most difficult task as people feel that by doing this they will be dishonouring the dead person in some way. There is often a feeling that to make moves towards a new way of life is betraying all that was most important to the individual before.

Recovery from bereavement is seen as a process of reconstruction, with new rules, different boundaries, changing relationships and some new behaviours.

This view of bereavement is therefore a positive one, dispelling feelings of helplessness by putting the bereaved person in control of their adjustment. The tasks that have to be accomplished may be facilitated by outside interventions when appropriate but it is the bereaved person who influences his own experience.

BEREAVEMENT AS A TRANSITION

A third perspective views bereavement as one of many life transitions, a transition being defined as 'a discontinuity in a person's life space' (Hopson and Scally, 1980). A transition is a major change, carrying the awareness that it is taking place and that one is expected to behave differently from before.

There are two main categories of change, those to do with personal development and those of major lifestyle, the latter being what concerns us here. It is pointed out that although we are now less likely to have to cope with the kind of transition that is caused by death, we are increasingly likely to meet other kinds of transition. Examples include frequent job changes, the possibility of periods of unemployment or redundancy, increased mobility and separation from family and a rising divorce rate.

They argue, therefore, that there are skills for coping effectively with these transitions, some people having more ability in this direction than others. If these skills can be identified and passed on to others it could help people to grow and develop from crises in their lives, rather than becoming demoralized and unable to cope.

Their approach is contained in a seven-stage model of the experience of transition or change and, like Parkes, they see this as a process, a sequence of events. These changes are centred on the self-esteem of the individual, on their perception of themselves. Although this approach is concerned with change rather than with loss as such, all change involves experiences of loss and therefore I find the work of Hopson and Scally (1980) can usefully be applied to bereavement (Figure 1.1).

Figure 1.1 A general model of the transition process (reprinted 1989 with kind permission of Hopson, B. and Scally, M., Lifeskills Associates, Leeds)

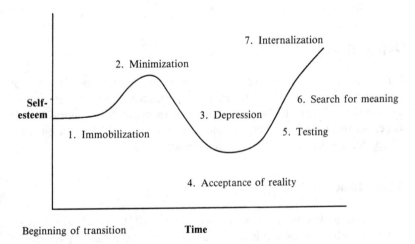

Immobilization

This may be seen as corresponding to the stage of shock and numbness described by Parkes (1972). The newly bereaved person is unable to mobilize their inner resources. The mind shuts off when forced to cope with severe stress, especially if this was not anticipated. We may liken it to the state of shell-shock known by soldiers in the First World War where they had to live for long periods in intolerable conditions, under constant threat of death. When the instinct for self-preservation was in conflict with duty it was possible for the individual to go into a state where he forgot who he was or what he was doing. In modern times, this may happen when the death was as a result of violence or a serious accident and the individual is paralysed with fear, immobilized by the stress they are undergoing. You may have, on occasion, observed a newly bereaved person appearing to show no emotion, but continuing to function competently at a practical level.

Minimization

This appears to be a form of denial. Sometimes it is expressed as an almost desperate desire to make the event less important, perhaps to feel that some control is being exerted over it. Bereaved people may make such comments as 'It's not as bad for me as it is for Mrs B over there!' (pointing to the wife of the patient dying in the bed opposite), or 'I know I'm luckier than some.'

Depression

The sadness that accompanies the realization of the finality of bereavement has been identified earlier. It is understandable that we may feel we should want to help the bereaved to avoid this uncomfortable stage, yet this avoidance may be due to a lack of confidence on our part rather than concern for the bereaved person.

Acceptance of reality

This is intimately related to the previous stage. All loss involves letting go which initially causes sadness and depression, yet no new patterns of living can begin until the reality has been faced and accepted.

Testing

This involves trying out the new self. There are new facets of the personality to be explored now that part of the old self is missing. There are different situations, new because the deceased person is missing from them. For example, someone who has been used to being part of a pair will have to face situations as a single entity. They will be treated differently by others whose perceptions will also have to change.

Search for meaning

There is usually an intense need to find some personal meaning in what has happened, and the very nature of bereavement seems to demand a think through or rethink of an individual's philosophy of living as well as their views of death itself. The Jewish psychiatrist, Victor Frankl (1963), writing of his experience in Auschwitz, quotes from Nietzche, 'He who has a why to live can bear with almost any how'. He describes how, in camp, when all the familiar goals of life were taken away and people suffered many kinds of loss, there still remained what he sees as the last of human freedoms, that is the ability to choose one's attitude in a given set of circumstances and, sometimes, to be able to rise above the outward fate. Bereaved people have a need to find their own meaning in what appears for most of them to be a meaningless and hopeless state.

Internalization

This is the final stage of the transition process. It is achieved when the individual has undergone change at a fundamental level. They have incorporated what has happened into their personalities, changed certain attitudes and have adapted to their changed pattern of living.

It can be seen, therefore, that these seven stages represent a cycle of major change with the disruption that it causes, gradually learning to acknowledge its reality, understanding the changed self and then changing behaviour and patterns of living. Finally, a balance is restored.

Transitions can be viewed as challenges, and positive as well as negative events may provoke similar reactions. The links between major changes and stress and illness is well recognized.

Holmes and Rahe (1967) devised a scale for measuring the seriousness of changes in people's lives (Table 1.1). The category for 'the death of a spouse' merits 100 units according to their classification, the 'death of a close relative' counting as 63. To put this into perspective, 'marriage' rates 50 units, 'pregnancy' 40 units, 'change of job' 20 units and, interestingly 'Christmas' is given 12 units! They consider that a total score of 300+ units in any one year was an indicator of a high likelihood of serious illness. Bereaved people are apt to score highly as many changes are usually associated with a death, for example moving house and/or changing occupation.

Table 1.1 The Holmes and Rahe social readjustment scales (reprinted 1989 with kind permission of Holmes and Rahe, 1967, Pergamon Press)

Units	Life event
100	Death of a spouse
73	Divorce
65	Marital separation
63	Detention – prison
63	Death of a close family member
53	Major personal injury or illness
50	Marriage
47	Made redundant or sacked
45	Marital reconciliation
45	Retirement from work
44	Major change in health/behaviour of family member
40	Pregnancy
39	Sexual difficulties
39	Addition to the family (birth, adoption, elderly person moving in, etc.)
39	Major business readjustment (merger, reorganization, bankruptcy etc.)
38	Major change in financial state (either worse off or better off)
37	Death of a close friend
36	Change to a new line of work
35	Change in number of arguments with spouse
31	Taking on a large mortgage
30	Foreclosure on mortgage or loan
29	Major change in responsibility at work
29	Son or daughter leaving home
29	Trouble with in-laws
28	Outstanding personal achievement
26	Partner begins or stops going to work
26	Beginning or stopping formal education
25	Major change in living conditions (extending, alterations, deterioration, etc.)
25	Change in personal habits (appearance, social life, etc.)
24	Trouble with the boss
23	Major change in working hours/conditions
20	Change in residence
20	Change in a new school
20	Change in recreation type/amount
19	Change in church activity (more or less)
19	Change in social activities
17	Taking on a small mortgage or loan
16	Change in sleeping habits
15	Change in number of family get-togethers (more or less)
15	Change in eating habits
13	Holiday
12	Christmas

It is interesting to note that both positive and negative life events feature on this scale. Between 60–80 is considered to be an average amount of stress. Above 100 you are at risk of the serious ill-effects of too much stress and need to take action to deal with that stress and to avoid, as far as possible, further stress in that year.

These three approaches show us different perspectives on what is a process of adaptation. This is enormously difficult, involving the modification of behaviour, expectations and self-definitions. It is far more than making the best of a bad situation, it is about change and the growth of human potential.

It also has to be realized that even when the bereaved person appears to be better, he or she may still suffer from recurring bouts of grief, usually long after everyone expects he or she to have recovered. C. S. Lewis (1961) writes 'One keeps emerging from a phase, but it always recurs. Round and round. Everything repeats. Am I going in circles?' The anniversary of a death and of other special occasions are also when mourning recurs.

In this chapter we have looked in detail at three approaches to the loss of bereavement. None of them should be looked at as being prescriptive, they are descriptions that provide us with insights to guide us and improve our understanding of the bereaved people for whom we care.

REFERENCES

Bowlby, J. (1961) Process of mourning. *International Journal of Psychoanalysis*, Vol. 42, pp. 317–40.

Caplan, G. (1964) *Principles of Preventive Psychiatry*, Basic Books, New York.

Frankl, Victor (1987) *Man's Search for Meaning*, Hodder and Stoughton, Sevenoaks.

Freud, Sigmund (1957) *Mourning and Melancholia, 1917*, Hogarth Press, London.

Gorer, Geoffrey (1965) *Death, Grief and Mourning in Contemporary Britain*, Cresset, London.

Holmes, T. H. and Rahe, R. H. (1967) The social adjustment rating scale. *Journal of Psychosomatic Research*, Vol. 11, pp. 213–18.

Hopson, B. and Scally, M. (1980) Lifeskills teaching programmes No. 1. *How to Cope with and Gain from Life Transitions*, Lifeskills Associates, Leeds.

Lewis, C. S. (1961) *A Grief Observed*, Faber and Faber, London.

Lindemann, E. (1944) Symptomatology and management of acute grief. *American Journal of Psychiatry*, pp. 101, 141.

Parkes, C. M. (1972) *Bereavement: Studies of Grief in Adult Life*, Penguin, Harmondsworth.

Pincus, Lily (1976) *Death in the Family: The Importance of Mourning*, Faber and Faber, London.

Worden, William J. (1984) *Grief Counselling and Grief Therapy*, Tavistock, London.

2. Culture, Customs and Rituals

Once people used to go to our cemeteries on Sundays and walk between the graves, singing beautiful hymns and spreading sweet-smelling incense. It set your heart at rest; it allayed the painful fears of inevitable death. It was almost as though the dead were smiling, from under the grey mounds. It's alright . . . don't be afraid.

Alexander Solzhenitsyn (born 1918)
(Reprinted with kind permission of the estate of
Alexander Solzhenitsyn and the Bodley Head)

INTRODUCTION

In our work as nurses, we are made aware of the multiracial dimension of modern British society and are likely to have experienced some of the ways in which culture influences the concerns of the patient and his family. It affects their needs and the kind of care and support they both expect and receive. It shapes beliefs about the causes of death and determines the ways in which the body of the deceased is treated and the ceremonies associated with its disposal. It also determines patterns and responses to grief and the role of the bereaved person. For example, bereavement may be organized around an effort to help the bereaved control themselves and forget the death, or be directed towards helping them express and live out their grief.

In sociological terms, the bereaved state indicates the status and role of the survivor of a death. In a typically small English family, for example, one in which the same few individuals fill most roles, the death of one (or more) leaves a great void. In the societies like the Samoans, households may contain many generations so that the acute trauma of bereavement is, to some extent, muted.

It has been suggested that we in Britain live in a society that is afraid of death, often to the point of denying its existence. Gorer (1965) analysed what he referred to as the 'pornography of death' in our culture. Instead of sex, death was the new forbidden topic. Most people reach maturity without ever seeing a dead person. Our expectations are that we, and those we love, will live until old age. The ageing process itself may be denied with millions of pounds being spent each year in cosmetics, hair colorants, plastic surgery and other ways of keeping the reality of gradual ageing at bay for a little longer.

However, another view is put forward in an *Observer* editorial (1980) which states:

> death is the media's new radical chic subject, fodder for endless TV programmes and newspaper articles. Bereavement, euthanasia, hospices – all have to come out of the closet and into the limelight. So can we still be a death-denying society? Though death may be a subject of intellectual debate, it is our most persuasive daily taboo.

Death has now come out of the closet, as it were. This may be as a result of a move towards a view of life as to do with personal growth. (see Rogers, 1961, for example). It may also be to do with a need for control and autonomy, a reaction against medical and technological power. Death is seen as all-powerful and is expressed in fiction, TV and videos, etc. as violence. It has been dramatized and, in this way, made more unreal.

D. J. Enwright (1983), the editor of the *Oxford Book of Death*, agrees with this view: 'I cannot say that I share the thanotologists' missionary urge to bring death out into the open. Much of the time, as a subject of conversation or even of solitary thought, it belongs elsewhere – standing to one side of life, which being so much shorter deserves to be given priority.'

In some other cultures, where natural death is a more common experience, an awareness of the transitory nature of life and an acceptance of death is encouraged. There are also guidelines as to how to behave and, as Walker (1982) suggests, although minority groups within our society may have a philosophy and rituals that seem strange to us, we can learn much from them.

In many such cultures, dying has meant moving up some kind of cosmological hierarchy, up into a world of gods or powerful spirits. The journey towards the afterlife might be fraught with dangers and ordeals of many kinds, so it is necessary to be familiar with this other world. It may be for this reason that many cultures that do believe in an afterlife have developed complicated and elaborate procedures to familiarize the dying person. An example of this kind of 'guidebook' is *the Tibetan Book of the Dead* (Evans-Wentz, 1980).

In our society we may believe that this approach encourages primitive fears in people who have been denied the benefits of structured, scientific knowledge. Our value system tends to reject an emphasis on the impermanence of life and labels such philosophies at the least as morbid preoccupations or, at worst, as signs of mental imbalance. Our medical system still tends to view the death of a patient as the ultimate defeat, reflecting the attitudes that the dying are losers in life's race. We tend to place high value on those with a 'fighting spirit'. The comment 'he fought until the end' is often made with pride by the bereaved family.

Indeed, death is seen as an adversary to be feared, fought and respected. This is one of the axioms of our culture. The surrounding mystery and controversy is of course unsurpassed, because nothing is more positively unique to each individual and at the same time more universal; it is the common denominator of mankind. Immeasurable time and energy has been spent trying to understand and come to terms with death, yet very few have succeeded in finding satisfying answers, in spite of information from many fields such as nursing, medicine, philosophy, religion, sociology, psychology, law, etc.

The ways in which the body may be disposed of are also of great significance to the bereaved person. Archaeology has established that from earliest times steps were normally taken to dispose of the body with appropriate ritual and respect, the living taking considerable risks in order to perform the necessary rites.

In modern societies, the lack of ceremony surrounding death appears to be detrimental to adjustment later on. Gorer (1965) suggests that greater suffering may be caused by the expectation in industrial societies for people to hide their grief and to control their feelings in public. Indeed, increasing number of deaths are 'hidden' in the sense that they take place in hospital and other institutions, away from the community.

Kalish (1977) points out that the behaviours surrounding death and bereavement are among those cultural features that are the 'most conservative and most resistant to change'. The funeral performs the necessary function of providing rules about how to behave and what is expected of all those involved.

THE FUNERAL

The word 'funeral' comes from the latin word *funeralis* which means 'a torchlight procession'. It is usually held within a few days of the death, and any delay, for example where a post-mortem and inquest has to be held or when the death is an unexpected one, can cause great distress to the bereaved person.

The funeral performs the practical task of disposal of the body and it serves as a ceremony at which relatives and friends can formalize their goodbyes. The letters of condolence, newspaper announcements, viewing the body and attending the funeral all serve to confirm the loss which, as we have seen, is the first step towards adjusting to it. These rituals are not isolated phenomena but are linked to the whole complexity of life experience within the context of a specific culture.

An example of this is provided by Ross (1981), writing about the Bakongo tribe of Zaire whose usual practice is to place the corpse on a rough wooden coffin and bury it, later erecting a cement gravestone. The widow of an American who had been buried in Zaire made arrangements that upon her own death her body would be cremated and her ashes deposited at her husband's grave. Since cremation is not practised by the Makongo the arrival of a container of ashes with their accompanying instructions provoked considerable consternation!

In the past it was customary for the body to be kept at home for a period but this occurs infrequently now. This direct contact with the deceased can be comforting to the bereaved although they may not ask for it at the time. The nurse in hospital or at home, who can gently and unobstrusively provide such an opportunity and offer support by her presence if this is wanted, is again helping the bereaved to accept the reality and to feel, when they look back, that they had the chance to say goodbye.

Expressing grief at this time and at the funeral does vary greatly between cultures. Some expect very open expressions of emotions and would feel that it was shameful and showed a lack of respect if such feelings were hidden. Europeans such as the Italians expect open emotional release, whereas our Anglo-Saxon culture tends to value those with strong emotional control.

It is also important to stress to relatives that their wishes, and any expressed by the deceased before death, can usually be put into practice – for example, the Polish family who wanted their mother to be fully dressed in her best clothes, in the coffin (apparently the usual practice in their culture), or the young man who asked to be buried with photographs of himself and his wife at their wedding, or the daughter who wanted her mother to be cremated wearing certain pieces of jewellery. (Special arrangements had to be made with the funeral director because jewellery is usually removed prior to cremation.)

In western society the usual practices are burial or cremation. Burial carries the very obvious and significant message that the body has returned from whence it came, back to nature, and there is a finality about viewing the coffin being lowered into the ground and throwing a handful of earth over it that emphasizes reality. The thought of being buried in the ground or having a loved one buried in this way can provoke many fears, and I have heard a number of bereaved people say that they would not want to face this particular ordeal. People also give very practical reasons for disliking this method, saying that they hate the thought of the graves being unnattended if they were not able to visit themselves.

Dying people may express the wish not to be buried for fear of this being a burden for the bereaved. My grandfather, when he was dying, said forcefully that if we buried him and then visited regularly with flowers he would get up and remove them!

Cremation is an increasingly popular method, being 'cleaner' and in some respects 'easier' for the bereaved to cope with. This notion of it being easier is often to do with the brevity of the ceremony which does not allow much time for absorbing its significance and because the coffin slides unobstrusively out of sight, thus the reality of which is happening does not always have its full impact on the grieving relatives.

However, the fact that there is no special place for the bereaved to visit when they feel the need may interfere with grieving. On the other hand, a permanent memorial can cause a bereaved person to feel guilty if they do not visit it regularly and so it could, arguably, prolong their mourning.

Providing those who wish it with ashes of their loved one to dispose of themselves may be helpful. It is not always easy even then, as Raphael (1985) points out, for the bereaved person to reconcile the ashes in their urn with the dead person. She quotes one person who said, 'He was such a big man. I cannot imagine him in that small box of ashes.' Conversely, a bereaved lady told me with some distress, of the very large bag of ashes she was given, which were of her mother. She took them to her favourite golf course and scattered them there but felt there were 'far too many' and suspected they included the ashes of someone else.

Research by Clegg (1988) into the decisions that bereaved people have to make found that religious reasons were rarely the basis for a choice between cremation and burial. The ownership of a family grave or the existence of a family tradition of burial seemed to be the main reason for choosing burial. Half the respondents chose what the dead person had indicated they wanted, 90 per cent had no regrets about their choice, but the other 10 per cent had varied regrets such as the actual choice of burial or cremation, not knowing where the ashes were, having no grave to visit or being unable to visit the cemetery or crematorium because of distance.

The wish for a memorial was commonly felt and this was often a headstone, or an entry in the Book of Remembrance. A rose, shrub, donation, plaque and seat were each mentioned by several people. The perceived helpfulness of a particular form of memorial was related to its connection with the dead person.

An important point made by Clegg is that as the main mourner makes the main decisions such as not to have a large funeral, not to have flowers, not to have a memorial, etc.; he or she may also be denying many relatives and friends an opportunity to grieve and say goodbye in their preferred way.

It is very helpful if they have discussed this together at some time in the past, because then the relative can follow the wishes of the person who died. Where this has not taken place, it is necessary for them to discuss the pros and cons with the funeral director, as it is the first decision that has to be made, affecting the number and types of death certificate that are required. It does appear that some bereaved people are helped by having a grave to visit although it could lead to over-preoccupation with the deceased. Similar comfort can be provided by having a special place in the relative's home or garden, where they feel they can communicate with the person who died. For example, many people plant a particular tree or rose in the garden as a memorial, others have a special corner of a room where they can have, for example, a photograph and a vase of flowers.

It is harder to let go and make a new kind of life when there is the commitment of a grave to visit, and it can be a source of worry to an elderly person if he or she is no longer fit enough to go. However, the trend is towards cremation and there is a garden of remembrance and a book in which the loved one's name is inscribed so that this can be viewed on, for example, the anniversary of the death. In many crematoria, the coffin is left on the plinth throughout the service and so, in a sense, it is the bereaved who have finally to take their leave from their loved one and this can be particularly hard to do.

Any kind of memorial to the dead person symbolizes the respect of the living and asserts a much needed belief that the memory of the dead person has not been entirely abandoned and that they will never be forgotten.

In some cultures, attempts have been made to preserve the body, presumably stemming from the belief in some kind of afterlife that will mirror the present one. Preservation of the body was intended to provide a permanent home for the spirit so that the personal identity was maintained.

There appears to be a small resurgence of this practice in our time, now that refrigeration can preserve a body indefinitely. The father of the trained nurse who died in the Middle East in 1980 under suspicious or unexplained circumstances fought a long campaign to find out what happened to her, and her body has been kept refrigerated for several years while this goes on. In the United States particularly, the practice of cryogenics has arisen where people can opt for their bodies or those of their loved ones to be kept frozen, presumably into posterity. A famous example is purported to be the body of Walt Disney which is kept refrigerated until a cure for the condition from which he died is found. This must surely be the ultimate example of denial of the reality of death to be found in our society today.

After the funeral ceremony is over, there is usually some kind of meeting together of family and friends with food and drink, which provides a valuable opportunity for the bereaved person to receive support and to feel a comforting warmth and concern. It is also cheering for them to be able to reminisce, sharing memories and experiences with others. It can help to renew and strengthen ties between family members, old friends and neighbours that may also be helpful in the longer term.

Although set ways of behaving are not rigidly laid down, it is generally assumed that the occasion will be a solemn one. However, this may not always be the case, notably of course the Irish wake. Jilly Cooper in her book *Class* (1979) describes how the whole family trooped home after the funeral (cremation) of her husband's grandmother and 'found crates of burgundy under the stairs. A riproaring party ensued and soon a lower middle class busybody who lived next door came bursting over to see if anything was wrong. Whereupon my father-in-law, holding a glass and seeing her coming up the path, uttered the immortal line "Who is this intruding on our grief?" '

Expressions of sorrow and laughter are often very close and many people wish their families and friends to dwell on happy memories. This is beautifully expressed by Joyce Grenfell (1980) in *Joyce: By Herself and Her Friends*:

If I should go before the rest of you
Break not a flower nor inscribe a stone
Nor when I'm gone speak of me in a Sunday voice
But be the usual selves that I have known.
Weep if you must
Parting is hell
But life goes on,
So sing as well.

THE ROLE OF THE FUNERAL IN HELPING MOURNING

(1) It provides an opportunity for self-expression. Nations throughout the world have different ways of meeting this. Some have professional wailers, the Irish have wakes, the Jews rend their garments – many forms of physical expression exist and most of these take place during the period of a funeral.

(2) The funeral provides the opportunity for communication. Individuals gather together during the funeral to express themselves to the mourners and the mourners can in turn comfort the bereaved by their presence. The bereaved should be encouraged to say the same things over and over again if they want to share memories and feelings. Sharing is inherent in the funeral process. The funeral is the combined effort of many. Grief shared is grief diminished, just as joy shared is joy increased.

(3) The funeral is a ceremony. Often survivors are numb after a death occurs, but the funeral arrangements must be made. These tasks and the presence of the mourners arouse the bereaved from immobility. They are kept busy and cannot withdraw. Unless there is a successful trend towards complete deritualization, there will always be some ceremony and this is often therapeutic.

(4) The environment can play an important role in the funeral. The provision of comfortable, convenient and beautiful surroundings can be comforting.

THE FUNCTION OF THE FUNERAL

(1) It provides an opportunity for the *manifestation of a shared loss* and a means by which the *support of the community* is conveyed to the bereaved. This gives a valuable sense of solidarity.

- It is an opportunity for public tribute.
- It is an expression of social understanding of the *relationship between the living and the dead.*
- There is the beginning of the process of *strengthening relational patterns* among those who survive.

(2) It assists in the *reinforcement of reality* for the bereaved.
(3) When the element of finality of death is conveyed there should be the eventual *freedom to develop new relational patterns* with the deceased. Thus it marks symbolically the end of one chapter and the beginning of another.

- It is an opportunity to release feelings and to say goodbye.

(4) The *religious and philosophical resources* for understanding and accepting death.

- *Meaning of life and death* must be presented in the light of the crisis of death.

Although most funeral directors are male there is a small, but growing number of females. Anyone can set themselves up as one, but reputable firms join the Association of Funeral Directors where membership is dependent on holding their diploma, and the premises are inspected regularly.

When caring for dying people of different faiths it may be tempting to assume that those who profess a certain religion (on a hospital record, for example) are in fact what they have stated, for example, a practising and believing Moslem or Jew. Neuberger (1987) emphasizes that 'it cannot be stressed too often that this is no more likely to be true than if someone puts "Church of England" down on the same form. It is quite likely to be merely a matter of labelling.'

She points out that for minority groups in western society, the issue is not only a religious one. Religious affiliation defines the community in which one lives, involving ways of living, grouping and distinction from other groups and marking the life-cycle changes of births, marriages and death.

When caring for patients and their families who are members of ethnic minority groups, their customs and religion must be considered sensitively. There may be special ceremonies that patient and family will want to be carried out and adjustments that can be made to hospital procedures (for example, the number of relatives who can visit at one time). Relatives may wish to express their grief in a particular way and a single room for the patient may also be very helpful. Ways of laying out the body and issues such as post-mortems, type of burial wanted, etc. need to be discussed. An interpreter is essential if the key relatives do not understand English well. Many patients and their relatives will find great comfort in turning or returning to the religion of their birth even though others may indicate that they no longer wish to practise it.

Nurses can help by refusing to join the general conspiracy fostered by our society that the death has not really happened. We can encourage the attitude that the funeral is not something, as many grieving relatives have put it, 'to be got through as quickly as possible' but an important way of showing respect and saying goodbye. As members of society we are aware that it is not only an individual concern but also affects the community in which that person lives. They need the support and understanding of that community which is a way of society sanctioning their right to grieve for what they have lost.

Gorer (1965) put forward the idea that the denial of grief in our culture goes a long way towards explaining the rise in violence and vandalism amongst younger people; work by Pincus (1976), Lake (1984) and others suggest that patients with psychiatric problems often have unresolved losses in their past.

Therefore, it is important that nurses do not avoid this subject out of misplaced anxiety or embarrassment about the belief that spiritual needs are not a nurse's concern. The nurse is in a position to meet these needs by her attitude of respect to the individual and their family, and by discussing those needs with the patient and family and bringing in the appropriate religious help with their consent.

In this chapter we have looked at some of the customs that have shaped our attitudes to death. We have looked at the rituals associated with the disposal of the body and emphasized their importance to the resolution of the grieving process.

REFERENCES

Clegg, Frances (1988) Crematorium, burial and memorials: the options and choices of bereaved people. *Bereavement Care*, Vol. 7 (2), Summer.
Cooper, Jilly (1979) *Class*, Eyre Methuen, London.
Enwright, D. J. (1983) (ed.) *Oxford Book of Death*, Oxford University Press, Oxford.

Evans-Wentz, W. (ed.) (1980) *The Tibetan Book of the Dead*, Open University Press, Milton Keynes.

Gorer, Geoffrey (1965) *Death, Grief and Mourning in Contemporary Britain*, Cresset, London.

Grenfell, Reggie and Garrett, Richard (eds) (1980) *Joyce by Herself and Her Friends*, Macmillan, London.

Kalish, R. A (1977) *Death and Dying: Views from Many Cultures*, Baywood Inc., New York.

Lake, Tony (1984) *Living with Grief*, Sheldon Press, London.

Neuberger, Julia (1987) *Caring for Dying People of Different Faiths*, The Lisa Sainsbury Foundation, Croydon.

Pincus, Lily (1976) *Death in the Family: The Importance of Mourning*, Faber and Faber, London.

Raphael, Beverly (1985) *The Anatomy of Bereavement*, Hutchinson, London.

Rogers, Carl R. (1961) *On Becoming a Person*, Constable, London.

Ross, H. R. (1981) Societal/cultural views regarding death and dying, *Topics in Clinical Nursing*, Vol. 3 (3): October.

Walker, Caroline (1982) Attitudes to death and bereavement among cultural minority groups, *Nursing Times*, Vol. 78 (50), 15 December, pp. 2106-9.

3. Family Needs: Before the Death of the Patient

I do not believe that any man fears to be dead, but only the stroke of death.

Francis Bacon (1561–1626)

INTRODUCTION

In this chapter, we are going to look at the role of the nurse in caring for the patient's family before death. Although most of the energy of the whole caring team is directed at the patient, the concept of total patient caring inevitably includes care of his family. The reasons for this are twofold. The enhanced confidence and calmness of the relative is both therapeutic to them and to the wellbeing of the patient. Awareness of the needs of the relative enables the nurse to see the patient as a member of a family group, understanding that he and his family are not separate entities but that each influences the other. Points to bear in mind include:

- The mental suffering of the family may be as great as the patient's.
- They may feel obliged to present a brave face and be afraid to reveal distress lest they make the patient feel a burden.
- They may find it difficult to take over the practical tasks and the responsibilities usually performed by the patient.
- They may appear callous, or at the least frivolous, if they try to maintain outside interest or social contacts.

- They may be so afraid to upset the patient that they avoid any contentious issue or any subject with meaning (this may, of course, be the pattern of a lifetime).
- They may feel a sense of failure if the patient dies in hospital, or dies without their presence if they wanted to be there.
- Their feelings may be ambivalent and they may feel guilty for not being loving towards the patient.
- Their reactions may mirror those of the patient. An example of this is provided by a study of 200 cancer patients and their relatives by Cassileth *et al.* (1985). There was a correlation between the scores for the patient–relative pairs – for example if the patient had high anxiety or depression, then the relative was likely to do so too.

In a recent review of bereavement studies, Lewis (1986) found some consistency in the relatives' expressed concerns. These were:

- fear of the future;
- feeling inadequate;
- anxiety about lifestyle changes;
- financial problems.

RELATIVES' NEEDS

Hampe (1975) researched into whether the spouse of someone terminally ill or who had recently died could determine their own needs. The spouses seemed to find nurses helpful to the dying patient but felt that they were too busy to help the families. The needs that the spouse identified in this study were:

- To be with the dying patient for as long and whenever they wished. A potential problem for nurses would be in balancing the needs of the patient against those of the relative. Sometimes patients need rest and protection from over-visiting.
- To be helpful to the dying patient and to care for their physical needs. Here it would be necessary to find out what, and how much, they felt able to do and to support them in this. Again their needs might not match those of the patients who may prefer that intimate care is performed by a nurse rather than a family member. As you may have experienced, it is also more time-consuming to teach and support someone else in that care.

- To be assured of the comfort of the dying patient by the competence and acknowledgement of health professionals. This gives security to relatives.
- To be kept informed of progress and of the plan of care.
- To be kept informed of the impending death of the patient.
- To be able to express emotion with others. This may be helpful for some relatives, but a word of caution: the availability of a member of the caring team needs to be assured, and they need to have both time and skills in order to be of use to the relatives. Parkes and Weiss (1983) pointed out how much easier it is to encourage the expression of emotion than to help it to end.
- To have comfort and support from relatives and friends.
- To have acceptance, support and comfort from health professionals.

INFORMATION

Another need expressed by the relatives in Hampe's study was for regular and detailed information. Hospitals have a reputation for withholding information and the following comments from a solicitor indicates the widespread feeling that a lack of information is a deliberate hospital policy.

> My father was admitted to hospital after a severe road traffic accident. I visited him every day but wasn't told anything. One day I walked into the ward to find his bed empty. He had been taken to theatre but no-one tried to contact me so that I knew what was happening. It might not be necessary when the patient is completely *compos mentis* but my father was an old man and confused at times and I wouldn't have thought he was fit enough to make those sort of decisions on his own. There were always different nurses. It seems it's pot luck who you are able to ask, sometimes. I felt that I was prevented from seeing those who made decisions. Each nurse I spoke to seemed to have a slightly different opinion, there was no 'official' information at all. I would have liked there to be one particular person who knew my father who was prepared to spend the time to talk to me, or even a department where one could go for information without feeling a nuisance . . . .

This man's experience highlights the feelings of frustration felt by relatives who cannot discuss the patient's progress as much as they wish. When major decisions have to be made, or grave information given such as the diagnosis after surgery, then the medical and nursing staff will usually seek out the relative in order to inform them. It would appear that the day-to-day progress report and explanation may be harder for the relative to find out and, indeed, they may feel they should not take up busy nurses' time by asking for this kind of discussion.

Nevertheless, experience suggests that this is often wished for and, once again, the provision of regular information helps them to feel they are involved and in control.

The implications for nurses of this study were the need to convey availability and time to relatives, the need to explain daily care, medications, tests, changes etc., and the need to listen to relatives' worries and current concerns.

This points to the need for good liaison between all the caring team, and communication with the patient and the family. Yet this is a problematic area. Stedeford (1981) states that 'communication problems cause more suffering than any other problem except unrelieved pain'.

VISITING TIMES

The first need in the list is of interest because it is one in which the needs of the relatives may be in conflict with the needs of the patient who may be easily exhausted by too much attention and company. Relatives may also value this facility but feel very guilty if they are unable to spend as much time with the patient as the hospital allows. It is an area that requires tact and diplomacy from the nursing staff. One way of giving both patients and relatives a break without the possibility of feeling guilty was introduced in the Christchurch Macmillan Unit where Mondays were reserved as non-visiting days. Of course dying patients were allowed to have visitors and exceptions were made using common sense. Otherwise the day was a peaceful one on which many relatives could catch up on practicalities and/or have a much needed rest while the patient could also have a break and did not feel neglected. It is easy, as you will have experienced, for such a patient to be over-visited.

The tie of visiting hours is well-expressed by this lady of 45, whose husband was ill for some weeks in hospital:

It's difficult when you go out to work, to be there at visiting times. At our local hospital they have visiting from 4 pm until 8 pm and as I have a demanding job I can't get there until 5.30 pm at the earliest, but even then it seems a long time until 8 pm. We soon ran out of things to talk about.

I wouldn't get home until after 8.30 pm and the next minute I'd have both his brothers on the 'phone long distance, asking the same questions again and expecting me to find out things for them. It was never-ending. When my husband was getting worse he was really quite difficult at times. Some evenings he didn't seem a bit pleased to see me, in spite of all the effort I'd made to get there. He stopped asking me about my life altogether and sometimes seemed cross with me – though I don't know of any reason – unless he felt I should have had him at home. But I couldn't have done that and keep my job.

This demonstrates the common problem of relatives who feel that they ought to be present at all the times allowed. It also points to the potential problems of asking that the close relatives be the key person to give out information to other family members. Although this may simplify communication problems for the staff and prevent the telephone lines being jammed by numerous anxious relatives and friends, it can add a considerable extra burden to the load carried by the key relative.

The following questions are helpful to consider before the death of the patient:

- With which family member will it be best to communicate?
- Do other members want to be involved/informed?
- Will there be any special customs or procedures that the patient and/or family will want to be carried out, particularly for last offices?
- What immediate support is likely to be needed by the family member? Can it be provided?
- Have the patient and family member been able to share the reality together?
- Does the family member want to be present at the time of death?

HOPE

Molter (1979) looked at what relatives perceived their needs to be and whether these were being met, and if so by whom. She found that relatives could identify their own needs during an intensive phase of hospitalization of their loved ones. The universal and strongest need was for hope.

What, then, are the implications for the care of relatives when this strongest need cannot be met? It is tempting for us and other members of the caring team to respond by making the kind of statements we know the relative wants to hear even if we word them in such a way that half-truths or veiled statements are expressed. Otherwise a commonly adopted defence is to avoid the relative as far as possible or to pass them ever onwards like a parcel from one to another - sister to houseman, houseman to consultant, consultant to social worker, social worker to sister . . . .

Yet even in this situation a positive approach can be adopted. Hope in terms of short-term goals for the patient and family can be encouraged. Looking forward to a day at home, a special meal, a visit from a valued friend, the achievement of sorting out a domestic problem can all contribute to patient and family feeling in control over what is happening to them.

I remember, for example, the relief (and incidentally, the reduction in analgesia) on the face of a patient with carcinoma of the lung when his wife was encouraged to leave his bedside in order to sort out a severe leak in the roof of their home. When she returned to the hospital having had it repaired (the kind of problem she had never tackled before) she had a quiet confidence about her which spread over the patient, leaving them both calmer than we had seen them before.

Hope can be provided in other ways. For example, the knowledge that the patient will not be allowed to suffer pain or great distress; the promise that someone will be with them when they are dying; the reassurance that the patient will be treated with dignity and respect; assurance that the relative will be involved and informed as much as they wish - all combine to give the feeling of being able to cope with whatever happens, thus helping to remove fears and worries about what the unknown situation will be like. Where it is possible to offer it, the knowledge that the relatives will receive outside help and support (if this is likely to be needed) also provides some security and hope for the immediate future.

Involving the relatives in all aspects of care of the patient, both physical and otherwise, is often discussed and it is generally agreed that, although this may initially be more time-consuming for staff, it may be beneficial in the long-term for patients and their relatives. In the situation of impending loss, this involvement may help to minimize feelings of guilt after the death. There is more likely to be a sense of accomplishment, of not having failed when one was needed, and a satisfaction of having done something tangible to show love and give comfort.

HOME OR HOSPITAL?

This is an important factor to be borne in mind when discussing the pros and cons of hospital versus home care. When being nursed at home is feasible because enough services are available and patients and relatives wish it, the family tend to feel a sense of achievement and pride when they have done so. Patients often express a desire to return to hospital because they are protecting their relatives who feel they would not be able to cope.

Woodhall (1986) looked at whether the terminally ill preferred to die at home or in hospital and found that the family played an important role. They tended to invest the professional with the responsibility of initiating discussion about this.

The main carer/family factors affecting this choice were:

- the carer's physical health;
- their emotional response;
- their ability to be a constant support;
- the existence of an extended family/friends support network;
- the age and sex of the carer.

On the other hand, relatives as well as patients may derive security from professional expertise and the certainty that any eventuality can be dealt with by a 24–hour hospital service. If, however, the relatives do not feel they are involved in the care and decisions concerning the patient, they may view the intimacy of the nurse/patient relationship with some anxiety, feeling helpless and threatened. As one old lady said to me, 'Those young nurses are always round the bend, fussing over him all the time. I hardly get a look-in, still he seems to like it . . . .'

INVOLVEMENT IN CARE

Relatives do indeed need to feel involved and may need much encouragement to give to the patient in any way they are able. Some may welcome the opportunity to help with nursing tasks if they are supported, others may prefer not to. The patient's wishes may be in opposition. They may prefer the nurses to perform intimate tasks, washing and feeding, feeling that it is undignified for these tasks to be done by a loved one.

A more active role for the relative may consist of bringing in special food or drink for the patient. I can recall a gentleman who, on the way to work each morning, called in with specially prepared grapefruit for his wife, presented with a cocktail of fruit on the top. Incidentally, he ended up supplying such grapefruit to the entire ward! It would have been possible for us to prepare something similar for her, but it was far more important for them both that he did it. Another gentleman adopted the habit of bringing in Chinese takeaways on many evenings as his wife could eat some of the rice dishes.

Others ways might include reading from a favourite novel, manicuring nails, arranging hair, ironing bedjackets or housecoats, redoing the flowers or bringing in special photographs to share. I am sure that from your own experiences you can add to this list, remembering that it can be important to point out some of these to an anxious relative who may not have thought of the practical things that seem so obvious to us. Doing practical tasks helps the relative to feel needed and in control and they are appreciated by the patient. It brings them closer together.

It is also important to help the relative to feel that sitting quietly by the bedside is still doing something that is needed. It can mean a great deal to be told that the patient, although apparently unconscious, may be aware of the relative's presence and find it comforting, and that this may be an opportunity to say the things they wish they had said, because the patient may still be able to hear and understand them. Throughout this time the nurse is there to act as the patient's advocate, balancing their needs and wishes with those of the relatives.

TIMESCALE

Expectations as to the timescale of a patient's last illness are of great concern to relatives who will often try to pin down the doctors and nurses as to definite time limits. Psychological adjustments are also made by the staff at certain stages, described by Strauss and Glaser (1968) as 'critical junctures':

(1) The patient is described as dying.
(2) Staff and family prepare for his death; the patient may also do so, if aware of his condition.
(3) It is felt that there is 'nothing more to do' to prevent death.
(4) The final descent – which may vary in length from weeks to hours.
(5) The 'last hours'.
(6) The 'death watch'.
(7) The death itself.

Strauss and Glaser also refer to the cause of dying as a 'dying trajectory' which takes place over time and can be plotted on a graph. Slow trajectories, particularly if longer than the relatives expected, can cause tension and guilt. The relatives may withdraw their support.

They refer to the 'awareness context' which is defined as 'what each interacting person knows of the patient's defined status, along with his recognition of others' awareness of his own definition'. They describe four kinds of awareness context:

(1) *Closed awareness* – where the patient does not recognize that he is dying, although everyone else around him does.
(2) *Suspected awareness* – when the patient suspects that he may be dying and tries to find out what his prognosis is.
(3) *Mutual pretence awareness* – where everyone knows the patient is dying, but all pretend that they do not.
(4) *Open awareness* – where the patient, his relatives and the staff all admit that death is inevitable and speak and act accordingly.

The appropriateness of an awareness context may be affected by the stages through which dying patients and their families may pass.

Stages of adjustment

Kubler-Ross (1970) determined that family members undergo stages of adjustment that are similar to the five phases she described dying patients going through; denial, anger, bargaining, depression and acceptance. She also states, 'We cannot help the patient in a really meaningful way if we do not include his family.'

She looked at death and dying long before it became in any sense 'fashionable' and, based on her work with dying children and adults over a ten-year period, she put forward a model of a process which they went through. These stages provide us with useful guidelines which can enhance understanding of patients who may otherwise be labelled as 'difficult'. However, they are not intended to serve as an end in themselves, I will use them as a framework on which to hang my experience of caring for patients and their families.

Denial
This is a very effective defence mechanism as we have already seen, and aptly described as 'selective forgetting'. The patient is faced with an

external reality – death – which is too unpleasant to face and so its existence is denied.

This can be so effective that a dying person may be unmoved by someone dying in the next bed because they do not believe it will happen to them. A very ill man in a four-bed ward where two others died in the night said, 'Well, I'm glad my time's not up yet!' Another said 'My X-rays and notes got mixed up with someone else's.'

Usually, denial is a phase, a buffer that 'buys' time while the patient mobilizes his inner resources to cope with reality. Paradoxically, it may be accompanied at times by a full realization of the truth, a subtle balance being maintained between acceptance and simultaneous rejection of reality. Is this easy to cope with? It can be difficult to know how to treat a patient who oscillates between these two extremes but, in spite of the fact that we operate under a climate of truth we also have to accept the right of the patient to put it aside whenever he wishes. ('Man cannot cope with too much reality.') Nothing will be achieved by trying to force reality on to an individual.

As the denial responses weaken, an isolating barrier may be felt by the patient between himself and the world outside. Expectations have to change, horizons must narrow. This growing sense of alienation leads to the emotions of the next stage.

Anger, rage and resentment

These are strong emotions. The question 'Why me?' is being asked, and also 'Why me and not *you*?' These are fundamental questions that no-one can answer; it is the individual himself who is being asked. We may find it difficult to say that we do not know the answer to these and similarly difficult questions.

This anger tends to be displaced all round the patient, the target moving from God, the doctor, other staff, the closest family and the dearest friend. Understandably, it can cause great distress to the recipient who usually has little to do with its cause. The patient may ring his bell frequently for apparently trivial reasons, be demanding of the staff's time and attention. Thus families and staff may wish to avoid him because of his aggressive behaviour.

Feelings of helplessness may add fuel to the rage. This anger may not be expressed directly. The introvert's outward calm may mask seething anger, which may be observed via facial expression and a rigid posture.

Bargaining

The anger subsides and the patient begins to consider the possibility of negotiating an agreement to postpone the end. For example, a possible bargain with God would be 'If I am good, I won't have pain.' With doctors an implicit bargain is often struck, 'If I agree to the treatment that you suggest, I will deserve to get better.' The natural longing to see some special event becomes mingled with the idea of receiving a prize for good behaviour. Mrs C said, 'I will endure anything if I can just live long enough to see my first grandchild born.'

Feelings of guilt may be associated with bargaining, especially where the cancer has been seen as a punishment for past behaviour, real or imagined. Mrs P, in her late thirties with two small children, expressed it to me as 'If I agree to have my mother-in-law come and live with us, as my husband wants me to, then I know I'll live to see my children finish school.'

The bargaining usually has a deadline included in it and the implicit promise that no further postponement will be asked, although this may not always be kept.

Depression

This is grief for all that is being lost to the patient. Many things must be left unfinished and usual ways of living, patterns of participation and giving to others have to change. There will be increasing physical dependence that cannot be denied.

This reaction to loss and deep disappointments of thwarted ambitions, frustrations, lost opportunities causes a withdrawal and sadness that has no easy solution and can make the family and the staff feel helpless. Everyone longs to *do* something to relieve this mental suffering. The family may need help to understand and to give the increased affection that is needed and to stay by the patient, otherwise this behaviour can further isolate him.

Acceptance

This is often seen as a goal for the patient. However, it may be inappropriate for some although it is undoubtedly easier for the family and for us. Kate Matthews (1988, and BBC2) said 'Little Nell may have died beautifully in a Dickens novel but I have no intention of going that way. I'll go out kicking and screaming . . . leaving a few ripples!'

For many patients, but not for all, this is the final stage. It may be a time when the patient feels life at its best, loved and cherished by those they care about, living life to the full within the constraints of the illness.

As interest in small details, in outside matters, diminishes the family may find this hard to understand. They may try to interest the patient at all costs, to hold his attention and keep him alive.

At this stage there can be a new significance of time and relationships and a heightened sensitivity to all that is beautiful. One lady said, 'I have never really lived until now – I live each moment to the full.' Psychologically, it seems that it is when we at our most vulnerable we are most willing to open up the doors of our personalities and expose our needs, given an environment that feels 'safe'.

As nurses, we have perhaps a unique opportunity here to ease this kind of situation enabling the patient and his family to make the most of it. If we are able to view this situation not as a failure but in a positive light, this will be conveyed to them and help them to do the same.

Armed with some knowledge of human behaviour during the stress of life-threatening illness, we may be able to understand our own reactions and approach the patient and his family in a helpful and therapeutic way.

The optimum way of learning is, of course, from the patients themselves. By having the courage to minimize the differences between 'them' and 'us' there is much they will tell which can benefit us both as nurses and people.

Kubler-Ross (1970) advocated that when there is time in which to do so, the family should be encouraged to express grief as much as possible prior to the loved person's death, and that this would to some extent alleviate the pain felt afterwards. Also, if different family members could share their feelings together this could facilitate later acceptance of it. That many families fail to share their feelings openly with one another when faced with this kind of situation may be due to the defence mechanism of denial and may also be a function of experience. Although we, as nurses, are being enlightened about combating this so-called conspiracy of silence surrounding death, it is also conceivable that some families have been overexposed to this viewpoint.

As Bowen (1978) pointed out, in spite of any attitudinal change that may be taking place 'the basic problem is an emotional one, and a change in the rules does not automatically change the emotional reactivity'.

Should nursing staff be closely involved with the family, sharing and supporting them and showing empathy by sitting and weeping with them? Kubler-Ross (1974) suggests that we answer this by asking ourselves how we would judge someone who cared enough to cry for us. But she adds, 'A display of emotion on the part of the therapist is like drugs, the right amount of medicine at the right time can work wonders.

Too much is unhealthy – and too little is tragic.' (We shall look more closely at the potential impact of this involvement for nursing staff in Chapter 10.)

She also suggests that if widowed people had been helped to bridge the gulf between each other when the partner was alive, then much of the battle to work through guilt and grief would have already been won.

TO TELL OR NOT TO TELL

This includes both sins of commission and of omission. Omission is when we do not provide the kind of supportive environment where the patient and family feel able to ask anything they want. Commission is when patients' questions are answered untruthfully or information is forced upon people who do not want to know. The foundation of trust between nurses, patient and relative, achieved via a gradual building of a good relationship, can, as you may well have experienced, be hindered or prevented by the dilemma of how much of the truth about the diagnosis and prognosis should be shared with the patient and, to some extent, the relative.

Decisions about whether to tell or not to tell have been, I think, appropriately rephrased by Melia (1987) as 'to lie or not to lie'.

In these difficult situations, which are part of the everyday experiences of many nurses, several people are involved. There is the patient, the key person in his life who may be a close relative or lifelong friend, the doctor, and always to some extent the nurse. As nurses we may often not be present when these matters are discussed but we are invariably involved in picking up the pieces, reinforcing, explaining or clarifying what was said or meant.

A central problem is to define what 'the truth' actually is. It is rarely a detailed analysis of the facts, few relatives or patients posing questions of the 'I have an isolated hepatic metastasis 2 cm in diameter, so what are the chances of recurrence in 5 years' time?' variety. Therefore, it is necessary to find out what the person is actually asking, rather than to make assumptions. One needs to know what the diagnosis actually means to them in terms of attitudes, expectations and past experiences.

An example of this from a patient's perspective was a single lady in her early sixties who had travelled the world as a musician and was found to have inoperable carcinoma. Each day she asked various nurses 'What is the problem? What should I be doing?' and she received back answers to the wrong questions, such as 'There is no problem for you at the moment, you must rest and let us do the worrying for you,' 'there isn't anything you have to do, let us do it for you'. After a few days of this, the charge nurse sat by her bed and asked her what exactly she wanted to know. Was she worrying about what might be wrong with her? 'Oh no,' she replied, 'that isn't very important. I am living in rented accommodation at the moment [having recently returned to England] and I want to know whether I should write to some estate agents and start looking for a flat to buy or whether this is not necessary'. The charge nurse told her that there was no need to do this at present. She seemed very content with this answer and died peacefully one week later.

The relative involved in this dilemma is very vulnerable and often expresses, at least initially, the wish that the patient be protected from the truth. This paternalistic desire to protect the patient from reality is often shared by medical and nursing staff. Relatives tend to describe their fears in terms of 'it will be too much for him', 'he will not be able to cope', 'he will give up', 'he might do "something silly" ', 'I know him better than you do, and he wouldn't be able to take it'. In all these statements there is likely to be some truth but they also reflect the fears of the relatives. If the close relative and patient have not had the kind of relationship where serious or threatening subjects have been freely discussed or deep feelings explored, it may indeed be hard, though not impossible, for them to begin to do so near the end of life. This can lead to collusion between doctors and relatives about withholding information and nurses can, often unwillingly, be forced into joining the conspiracy. However, because of the amount and quality of daily contact between the nurse and patient and relative, it may often be the nurse who can help a relative to see the advantages of being open and honest with the patient when and if the patient wishes it, and offer moral support to the relative who feels insecure and overwhelmed by the situation.

An example of this problem was a couple in their fifties who were being visited at home by their general practitioner and community nurse. Each day the husband asked the nurse to tell him what was wrong and whether he would recover or not. At the same time the wife would ask her if she had told him anything. 'If you do,' she threatened, 'I won't have you in the house again. I know my husband and he would turn his face to the wall and give up. He doesn't want to know really. And I can't bear to talk about it.'

It took many days of gentle discussion and questioning for the wife to be able to admit to her own fears – 'I wouldn't know what to say, I wouldn't know what to do, *I* would give up'. It also took time to convey the reassurance that nothing would be said to her husband that he had not specifically asked to know. The eventual outcome was the breaking down of the barriers and false atmosphere that had pervaded the house before, and some weeks of closeness between them before his death. Afterwards, his wife told the community nurse that those weeks had been the closest of their married life and that they were a comfort to her to look back on.

Even where there has been an open dialogue between patient, relative, doctor and nurse there are likely to be some differences. For example, the information is usually couched in more optimistic and hopeful terms when given to the patient than to the relative.

Relatives tend to be very persistent about being given some idea of the prognosis of the patient. Many doctors, and sometimes nurses, have been pushed into giving time limits and these are noted very carefully by the relative. It is not unusual for the days to be marked off on their mental calendar, causing much distress. It can lead to the patient being overprotected by being left out of family decision-making. There may be also be difficulties if the patient outlives the given prognosis time because this period is seen as being finite, and they have gathered their resources to carry them through. If the patient then outlives this time-limit and perhaps begins to improve, there may be confusion and feelings of frustration or irritation about which the relatives feel very guilty. If past relationships have been unhappy then these feelings can lead to rejection of the patient.

Lucien Israel (1980) asks us if the choice is between truth and charity. The conflict that we, as nurses, experience, is between our responsibility as the patient's advocate with its underlying value of the patient's right to self-determination and autonomy. He has the right to the amount and quality of truth that he feels he needs. At the same time there is the assumption of authority by the patient's doctors, on the paternalistic grounds of being in some way 'better' for the patient.

Ryan (1979), describing a study carried out in Russia, quotes a distinguished Russian professor who was defending the view that patients should not be told the truth, informing the patient of the diagnosis 'does not mobilize the will – it paralyses it'. A patient who is ignorant of his condition 'will recover more rapidly, after which he will have peace of mind and will not live in fear of the illness returning'. Many of us have come across this approach.

Sometimes nurses feel trapped between patient, relative and doctor, and need to explore carefully their own feelings and to have the courage to act as the patient's advocate, when this is needed, to improve communication and, therefore, understanding between all involved. When this can be achieved it provides a solid foundation of trust and security for the relative as well as the patient, and it may also greatly improve the quality of the remaining life together.

A family's burden may be exacerbated by not understanding what the dying patient may be going through at this time. This is well-explained by Hinton (1968):

> 'The dying often find the settling of various practical matters concerning family life, property and work responsibility a satisfying task. They can get a sense of completion. . . . They can take plesure in ensuring that their dependents will be grateful for the forethought. Sometimes, those who are aware that their existence is to be curtailed, may get a little more from life by advancing, bitter sweet though this may be. It is not uncommon for dying people to get more pleasure out of these remaining days than others would believe possible. . . . Other people when dying will not want to do things but can quite pleasurably review their life, on the whole satisfied with its achievements and satisfactions. Some, knowing the situation, will wish to prepare themselves spiritually for the anticipated eternal existence.

I know of several examples from my own experience, of families who told me that these last weeks or days were the closest and happiest of their lives. This should always be borne in mind and I suggest that the nurse has a role in interpreting the wishes and needs of the dying patient to the relative, to prevent misunderstandings that can mar the last times they have together. For example, the lady who did not understand her sister's appearance of contentment and her declining interest in their usual concerns interpreted this as meaning that her sister did not really love her and so did not mind leaving her. A staff nurse taking time and trouble to explain what the patient might be feeling and why, and her encouragement to the sister to talk openly about this altered their last few days and left the sister with happier memories to look back on.

It has been suggested that the vulnerability of the relatives is due in part to the fact that when adults are in serious trouble their emotions tend to regress. We become more childlike and look to authority figures for comfort and security. We may appreciate more physical contact than usual. Where appropriate, physical comfort such as an arm round the shoulder or holding a hand can be valuable.

Throughout this discussion of the needs of relatives before the death the role of the nurse has been emphasized. However, it must be remembered that the nurse is not the only member of the caring team who is able to help and may not always be the appropriate person to support a particular relative at a particular time. When time and resources are short, it may be appropriate for others to be involved in caring for the family although it is often the nurse who immediately comes to mind. It may also be possible at the right moment to instigate support between different relatives of ill patients on the ward or to involve volunteers, suitably supported, to provide caring listening and comfort. Depending on their involvement, many others may be able to help – for example the physiotherapist who is treating the patient, the specialist colostomy nurse who is advising them, the liaison sister or health visitor who may be involved in helping the relative to go home even if for a very short period. Any person who knows the patient will be able to give valued information and discussion with the relative if this arrangement is made.

Writing in 1981, McNulty put forward some of the problems nurses face in trying to meet the needs of the relatives:

> Nurses have a lot to answer for in their apparent insensitivity to the needs of relatives . . . . I think that we are sometimes afraid to stop for fear we might not be able to answer the questions asked, afraid because we cannot give the so much wanted good news, afraid because we might have to say 'I don't know'. If only we could realise that just by stopping for a moment and sharing our presence, we may have to some degree lightened the family's burden.

In this chapter we have looked at the patient and his family as a complete unit, knowing that our care of one is likely to have a beneficial effect on the other. We have considered the difficulties that may arise in trying to meet the needs of the patient and those of his family. We have also discussed what, when and how we should answer the patient's and relative's questions.

REFERENCES

Bowen, M. (1978) *Family Reactions to Death in Family Therapy and Clinical Practice*, Aronson, New York.
Cassileth, B. R. *et al*. (1985) A psychological analysis of cancer patients and their next of kin. *Cancer*, Vol. 55, pp. 75-7.
Hampe, S. (March, April 1975) Needs of the grieving spouse in a hospital setting. *Nursing Research*, Vol. 24, p 2.
Hinton, John (1968) *Dying*, Penguin, Harmondsworth.
Israel, Lucien (1980) *Conquering Cancer*, Penguin, Harmondsworth.
Kubler-Ross, Elizabeth (1970) *On Death and Dying*, Tavistock, London.
Kubler-Ross, Elizabeth (1974) *Questions and Answers on Death and Dying*,

Macmillan, London.

Lewis, F. M. (1986) The impact of cancer on the family: a critical analysis of the research literature. *Patient Education and Counselling*, Vol. 8(3), pp. 269–89.

Matthews, Kate (1988) A fight to the death, *The Times*, 27 October.

McNulty, Barbara (1981) *Problems Related to Death: Care for the Dying. Final Report*. European Public Health Committee, Strasbourg.

Melia, Kath (1987) Everyday ethics for nurses: to lie or not to lie. *Nursing Times*, Vol. 83(3), pp. 30–2, 21 January.

Molter, N. C (1979) Needs of critically ill patients, a descriptive study. *Nursing Research*, Vol. 8(2).

Parkes, C. M. and Weiss, R. S. (1983) *Recovery from Bereavement*, Basic Books Inc., New York.

Ryan, Michael (1979) Ethics and the patient with cancer. *British Medical Journal*, Vol. 2, pp. 480–81, 25 August.

Stedeford, Avril (1981) Couples facing death. *British Medical Journal*, Vol. 17, p. 283, 17 October.

Strauss, A. L. and Glaser, B. G (1968) Patterns of dying, in Cox, C. and Mead, A. (eds) *A Sociology of Medical Practice*, Macmillan, London.

Woodhall, Chris (1986) A family concern. *Nursing Times*, Vol. 82(42), pp. 31–3, 22 October.

4. Family Needs: At the Time of the Patient's Death

The hour of departure has arrived, and we go our ways – I go to die and you to live. Which is the better, only God knows.

Socrates (469–399 BC)

INTRODUCTION

There would seem to be no single suitable definition of death; at best we can only describe it. It can be a series of gradual losses and is therefore as complex and extraordinary as individuals themselves. As expressed by Kalil Gibran, 'If you would indeed behold the spirit of death, open your heart wide unto the body of life. For life and death are one, even as the river and the sea are one.' But when does the river become the sea?

Defining when death actually takes place is becoming increasingly complicated for nurses and doctors alike. It is rarely instantaneous, neither is it a single event. In biological terms death is a process, occurring in stages, and there are variations in the rate at which the final point is reached.

Final death is merely the last in a series of functional, organic, and partial deaths because although the organs coexist together, they die separately from one another. Indeed, the day of our birth is one day's advance towards our death!

SOCIAL DEATH

As nurses, most of us will have come across what is known as *social death* – for example, when an elderly person is admitted to a long-stay ward, or moved to a rest home or nursing home, or even when they have moved on retirement to an area where they know few people, and their partner dies. A retired gentleman living alone who had congestive cardiac failure described his situation to his community nurse by saying it felt as though 'I'm dead already'. A bereaved person may be left with little or no contact with family or long-term friends, and may be isolated and removed from the daily contacts which most of us take for granted. We may also have had experience of disabled or mentally handicapped people being treated by others as if they are not present, and their opinions and needs are not considered. This attitude is summed up for me by the apt title of the Radio 4 programme for the disabled, 'Does He Take Sugar?'

PSYCHOLOGICAL DEATH

For some people retirement produces 'psychological death'. People for whom the world of work has provided not only their *raison d'être* but their friends and pattern of living suffer a loss of identity when they retire because their self-image is tied up with their work role. They are unable to make plans for a future they cannot envisage and they may feel abandoned by those who are important to them. This ending of relationships and loss of a role can cause deep depression so that the individual does, indeed, seem to be psychologically or emotionally dead.

BIOLOGICAL DEATH

The most difficult problems of definition occur with biological death. An example of this is quantifying what is meant by a 'terminal illness'. I have asked many different groups when they consider that someone is terminally ill and the answers vary greatly. Some see the answer in numerical terms, perhaps six months, six weeks or six days. Others see this beginning with physical loss such as being confined to bed or needing help with certain activities of daily living. A few put forward the view that this begins from the moment the patient realizes he may not recover (whether he has been told this or not), or else it begins when and if the patient's will to live becomes weakened and he no longer fights for survival. Usually one person in the group will point out that we are all terminally ill, in other words we start to die from the moment we are born! In the critical care area, biological death may not be considered to have happened until life support equipment has been disconnected and even then, as vital signs are observed, total death may be delayed for some time afterwards.

ANTICIPATED DEATH

The acknowledgement that the dying person has special needs and rights is not a modern phenomena; for centuries compassion and consideration was given to the dying, and a principal function of nurses was to provide the necessary comfort at this time. It seems likely to have been the advent of the medical model, holding out a promise of curative treatment to the majority, that changed the focus of nursing from care to cure. Most of us are able to accept that, for some patients, active treatment may become inappropriate, and dilemmas over the role in livesaving measures (in certain cases) are frequently voiced.

The hospice movement, with its emphasis on support for patients and their families and its research-based methods of symptom control, has had a worldwide influence on the care of dying patients, particularly since the opening of St Christopher's Hospice, Sydenham, in 1967. The Macmillan Units and domiciliary care services, whose capital costs were met through the National Society for Cancer Relief, started with the Christchurch Macmillan Unit and Home Care Programme in 1975, with a similar philosophy and aims. By their very existence they brought the special needs of those who were dying to the attention of nurses and other health professionals. This care always included consideration of the needs of the patient's family. Their philosophy accepted the reality of death but, very importantly, put forward to the medical and nursing professions the idea that each patient is living, not dying, until the end.

The problems for the dying person and his family of being cared for in a manner suitable for their own unique situation was highlighted by the European Public Health Committee Report (1981):

> Considering that in our society a man dies badly if neither he nor his family accept the fact of dying; a man dies badly if the medical team is unaware of the problem, untrained to deal with them and not in control of the situation; a man dies badly if death is relegated to the realms of the

irrational, the imaginary, the terrifying; a man dies badly if he dies alone in a society which no longer knows how to die.

Perhaps another reason for dying badly in our society is that the family have not been involved as much as in the past, in part due to the tendency towards hospitalization.

As Aries (1974) put it:

> Today the initiative has passed from the family, as much an outsider as the dying person, to the doctor and the hospital team. They are the masters of death – of the moment as well as the circumstances of death – and it has been observed that they try to obtain from their patient 'an acceptable style of living while dying'. The accent has been placed on 'acceptable'. An acceptable death is a death which can be accepted or tolerated by the survivors.

But what about these survivors? What are their needs likely to be at the time of death? Earlier I put forward the view that one cannot isolate the needs of the family from those of the dying patient because their reactions contribute to the patient's view of himself and his situation. It is usually the nurse who will try to meet these needs as she is in constant attendance and usually perceived by them as being the most approachable professional.

Therefore, it is a nursing responsibility to assist the family to cope successfully with the difficulties of caring for the patient, at the time of death. It is feasible that the way the relatives are supported could have a profound effect on their adjustment to bereavement after the death. Perhaps a useful framework is to consider the needs of the relative as we do those of the patient, dividing them into physical, psychological, social and spiritual needs.

PHYSICAL NEEDS

The physical needs of the family appear to be a minor concern when their loved one is dying, whether this lasts for hours or even for a few days. At one time or another I am sure we have all urged the family to go away for a while and rest or to leave and have something to eat, and we have provided hot drinks or made them a snack, probably as much to demonstrate our caring attitude in these circumstances as to meet any kind of physiological need. Where it is possible to provide a bed or easy chair for a relative to stay by the bedside overnight, this too conveys warmth and involvement to the relative.

Reflecting back on my own practice I wonder if, on occasion, it is possible to consider physical needs at the expense of emotional ones? The relative who may be exhausted and drained at the time of death from having given everything they can, later has the satisfaction of having done so. It may be that this can give much greater long-term relief to the bereaved person.

The nurse's role here is to support, encourage and show she has confidence in the relative's ability to succeed. Like other self-fulfilling prophesies, this expectation that even the most anxious and isolated relative will be able to stay and share with the dying patient can go a long way towards ensuring this outcome.

Of course, not every close relative does want to be present at the death of their loved one. This may be because they have witnessed a death in the past that was unpleasant or undignified, they may fear that they would be unable to cope or they may not feel close to that person. It is necessary to find out what they really feel and accept them as they are that moment, respecting their right to do as they wish. It follows that the nurse must also support their decision afterwards.

A more difficult situation arises when the relative wants to be with the patient but does not get there in time, one of the many problems of sudden death or deterioration. Then it is essential for someone to spend time with them to allow them to express their feelings and be able to tell them what happened.

This often needs reinforcement and it is necessary to offer the relative the chance of coming back to the ward or department or of receiving a later visit from the community nurse, so that events can be gone over again and again until the relative has assimilated them. A picture of what happened is thus formed in the relative's mind, and the reality is likely to be easier to bear.

Many of us have been put in the difficult position of deciding to advise the relative to have a break for a few minutes, feeling certain that the patient will die while they are absent from the bedside. It seems as if in some way the strength of the relative's need and will to keep their loved one with them, delays the death happening. If the relative is not present the knowledge that someone else was with the patient when they died, so that they were not alone, may be comforting.

In all these circumstances, the nurse has a great opportunity to give support and comfort, assisting the family to cope with the unknown and in doing so they often find strengths of which they had been unaware.

PSYCHOLOGICAL NEEDS

The psychological needs of the relative cannot always be separated out. The emotional nature of their last time with the dying patient may colour their perception of events, and this must always be borne in mind by nurses and other carers.

There is, for example, a need to explain medical and nursing procedures near the end of life because these can sometimes be misunderstood at the time or cause puzzlement when later reviewed. The relative may be too upset or too polite to ask for explanation at the time, and as nurses we may make assumptions about their knowledge and understanding that may prove erroneous.

One example that may cause distress is when the patient is semiconscious and it seems no longer appropriate for them to eat. Some relatives as well as patients are relieved to find that food is no longer being encouraged, while others may see this as a form of neglect or an abandonment of any attempt to improve or cure their condition. Another example is the giving of medication very near the end. A repeat injection of analgesia to ensure the patient's comfort, or of hyoscine to dry up the secretions, may be misconstrued by the anxious relative waiting outside the screens, particularly if death takes place shortly afterwards. Even routine nursing care that takes place near the death may become linked to it in the relative's mind.

These nursing situations merit explanation before as well as afterwards, so the relative may feel comforted by the consideration given to them and not mystified, or unintentionally misled as to what has been done and why.

It is often pointed out that relatives need to express their feelings at this time, and it is important to do all we can to provide privacy for them and the time to remain with the body after the death in order to say goodbye in their own way.

The encouragement of the expression of emotion to nursing and other staff needs to be thought through carefully. There are many demands on time and resources, and if we actively encourage expressions of grief we must be able to carry it through not offering what in reality we cannot give. It is obviously critical that when they leave us in hospital, or when we leave them at home, we have helped them to bring themselves together again, and hopefully to be feeling some relief from sharing their feelings with us.

It is of interest that in a piece of nursing research conducted by Freihofer and Felton (1976) it was shown that the four nursing behaviours most *disliked* by the relatives of dying patients were:

- encourage me to cry;
- hold my hand;
- cry with me;
- remind me that the patient's suffering will soon be over.

In meeting psychological needs, the nurse's role is to give practical advice and information, to put relatives in touch with other members of the caring team who may be of help to them, and give them supportive warmth and caring concern (see Chapter 10 for the skills needed).

Social

Social needs can be viewed as a need to share experiences and to feel part of a community. Often the very situation the grieving relatives are going through isolates them from their usual way of life, friends and networks. It is sometimes possible to introduce or encourage the forming of a relationship between different relatives in a ward or in a small community that can help to relieve isolation and provide opportunities for the sharing of experiences. It may also be helpful to encourage the relative to accept help of any kind from family, friends or neighbours. This may be refused by the relative who wants to be seen by everyone as being able to cope.

Relationships are often far from straightforward and this can mean that there may be rifts between family members, people who are important to the patient may be missing or estranged, and emotional battles may be going on between relatives. It is uncommon, but not rare, in my experience, for arguments to actually take place round the bedside of the dying patient.

When death is anticipated, it provides the patient and family with an opportunity to heal old wounds, to tie up 'loose ends' and to explain their feelings in ways they may not have tried before. People who have not seen each other for many years may come together at this time.

An even more difficult situation met with occasionally is when the dying patient has been involved in more than one close relationship. A classic example of this was a gentleman in his fifties dying of advanced cancer who had both a wife and a mistress who loved him. Much sensitivity to the wishes of all three were needed in order to arrange that he spent time alone with each of them and that they did not meet. It was also very important to realize that the mistress was likely to be left with little sympathy or support in her loss that was going to be for her a 'hidden' bereavement.

There is a need for privacy both at the time of death and after it, yet in many wards and departments a private room does not exist.

Close liaison with the medical social worker is necessary and helpful when trying to meet the social needs of the patient and family.

Spiritual

Many nurses feel out of their depth when spiritual needs are considered and this may be because there is often confusion between spiritual and religious needs. All of us have a spiritual dimension, it is part of the whole person, and many patients and relatives turn or return to some kind of religious beliefs at this time.

Whatever the patient's or relative's beliefs, the offer of a blessing to be said for them before and after the death can be very comforting and rarely refused. Others find their faith or philosophy of life is being severely questioned, perhaps for the first time. Either way, the search for meaning inevitably raises many questions and a desire to think or talk through ideas. The nurses can refer a patient or relative to the chaplain or local vicar or priest and the suggestion, if done tactfully, can be very welcome. There is an understandable reluctance to bring up this subject, yet it is rare for the suggestion to be objected to, even if the relative declines the opportunity. Experience also suggests that even where families are anxious to protect the grieving relative from callers, the local minister's arrival on the doorstep is welcomed as someone who will have some help and comfort to offer. Ainsworth-Smith and Speck (1982) point out that even those who have abandoned religious observances of any kind still tend to hold expectations of the clergy and that, in this sense, the clergy represent the longings of others and are vested with a reverence and respect.

Longbottom (1986) conducted a survey among his fellow clergy and a number of bereaved people and found that, on average, clergy were faced with a funeral every nine days, and one that left a widow or widower every seventeen days. He found that, while most gave high priority to contact with widows and widowers before the funeral, a large number ceased to have any contact after it. Time, therefore, might well prevent follow-up support but, as he suggests, assistant ministers (for example, curates, retired clergy, etc) or lay members of the congregation could be used. There was great scope for compassion. My own experience of visiting bereaved people seems to bear this out, and I found a number of them who expressed the wish that the clergy would visit them again.

The clergy are presented with an immense opportunity in relation to bereavement, which, Longbottom found, was only being taken up by a small number. He points out that the bereaved are likely to be feeling numb at the funeral and unlikely to remember the majority of what is said. He suggests that the clergy and the bereaved often have different aims, the clergy being trained to use the opportunity to proclaim Christian truth, while the bereaved tend only to recall what was said about the deceased and statements of thanksgiving for their life. His view is that there is a need for the clergy to be more involved after the funeral when the bereaved are likely to be more receptive to discussion and comfort derived from the Christian perspective.

I found a number of bereaved people who, once family and friends had started to withdraw their presence and many of the practicalities had been dealt with, expressed the need to talk about their philosophy of life and welcomed contact with the clergy. Wherever possible I arranged this, with their consent, or actively encouraged them to do so themselves. I had to overcome my own initial reluctance to be involved, feeling that attention to spiritual needs was, in some way, different from other needs, and that concern could easily become undue interference. Each of us, as nurses, have to decide what our role should be in this respect but I suggest that it is part of our function to be concerned with spiritual needs, provided we do not impose our own views over the expressed wishes of the relative.

THE FUNERAL DIRECTOR

Part of the caring team at the time of death is the funeral director. He offers an emergency service, working intensively during the initial crisis and, unlike most other carers at that time, provides very personal help to someone previously unknown to him. His ability competently to guide the newly bereaved person can do much to disperse feelings of helplessness, and the qualities of gentleness, friendliness and tact are very much needed at that time. A good funeral director is, therefore, a valuable member of the team and the nurse may, on occasion, be asked to recommend one to relatives. If so, it is obviously necessary to be conversant with hospital or local authority policy but, within their guidelines, there is often scope to steer a distressed family towards one who has been found to be efficient and caring.

Relatives who are concerned about the cost can be encouraged to obtain more than one estimate. Since the abolition of the £30 death grant, people who are on supplementary benefit can, depending on the amount of their savings, have part or all of the funeral costs paid for by the DHSS. Only one estimate has to be produced and what is referred to as a 'decent, simple funeral' can be entirely paid for. (When the deceased person is destitute the hospital or local authority are bound to pay for a simple funeral for them.) It is also important for relatives to consider carefully what their priorities are so that they have the kind of funeral they wish.

It is necessary for the nurse to make contact with the chosen funeral director as soon as possible after the death so that the essential practical details can be dealt with, even though the interview with the relatives can take place much later, if they wish. Figures 4.1 and 4.2 and Table 4.1 show the practical considerations to take into account when discussing funeral arrangements.

Table 4.1 What has to be done after the funeral (although not necessarily in this order)

Claim state benefits
↓
Pay undertaker
↓
See solicitor to discuss the will of the deceased; wind up estate
↓
Answer letters and thank for flowers
↓
Choose memorial stone and order stone masons (if required)
↓
Arrange memorial service (if required)

Nurses who have been closely involved with a dying patient and his family may be invited to attend the funeral. It is, of course, an honour to be asked to do so and nurses may feel they have to agree even though it may be at a difficult time or make emotional demands upon them. Specialist Macmillan and hospice nurses may find this happening very frequently. It is important to learn how to refuse gracefully and without guilt when it is appropriate to do so.

It is apparently not uncommon for a relative to contact the funeral director before an expected death takes place, in order to set their minds at rest on a particular point and this may be seen as being part of the process of anticipatory grief previously described.

Figure 4.1 What has to be done when the patient dies. (Reprinted from *What to Do When Someone Dies*, with kind permission of the Consumers' Association)

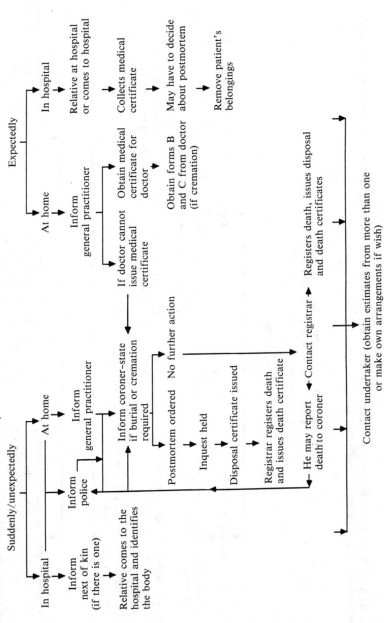

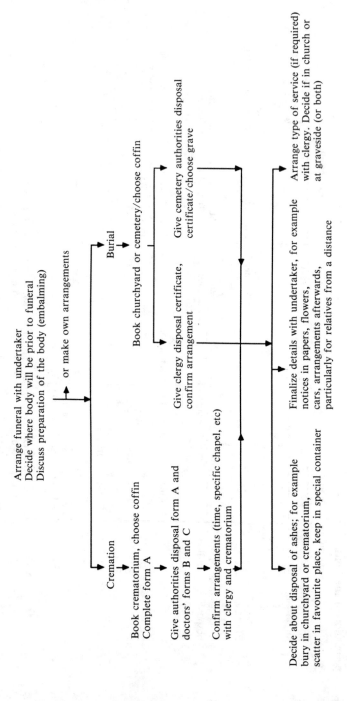

Figure 4.2 What has to be done to arrange a funeral. (Reprinted from *What to Do When Someone Dies*, with kind permission of the Consumers' Association)

SAYING GOODBYE

It can be comforting for the relative to be able to visit the chapel of rest and sit with the body of their loved one. Although in this country elaborate preservation of the body is not made unless specifically requested, it is the usual practice to do a form of embalming in order to enhance appearance.

It may provide a much-needed opportunity for the bereaved person to say goodbye and express their feelings to them for the last time. It is also a valuable opportunity for others who were close to the person who died but not with them at the end. It may be appropriate for the nurse to point out this possibility, particularly when the death took place in surroundings where privacy and dignity are difficult to preserve, such as the intensive care or accident and emergency departments.

Wright, Cousins and Upward's (1988) report on bereavement support in NHS hospitals in England is based largely on the personal experiences of those whose relatives and friends died in hospital. It provides, as Hempel (1988), points out, 'harrowing examples of callousness among individuals and organizations whose entire rationale is supposed to be caring'.

Hempel's news report alerts us to the special problems of those who are bereaved while they, themselves, are hospital patients. She poignantly describes the plight of a lady who was paralysed in a car crash which injured her husband and son and killed her daughter. She was informed of her daughter's death while lying in a ward full of psychogeriatric patients. Her suggestion that her daughter's body be brought to her was greeted with horror. She was taken to casualty and had to say goodbye to her in a room full of strangers. She later learned there had been a row because the nursing officer had objected to her seeing the body.

Polly Bird (1986), writing in the *Guardian*, shares her personal experience of what she calls 'the overwhelming need to look death in the face':

When I was in my final year at college, my boyfriend was killed in a car crash. At least that's what I was told and had to believe, because I never saw the body.

A young policeman called in the middle of the night. A photo of a girl had been found in my boyfriend's jacket and a girl lay dead between the two cars involved. He had to check to see if it was me. It wasn't, of course; the girl had been thrown from the other car. He was then extremely distressed at having to break the news to me.

My friends in the block were told and valiantly sat with me through the night while I wept. The college sister gave me a tranquillizer. A friend of my boyfriend drove me to the cremation ceremony. There we watched a coffin disappear into flames. Even now I find it difficult to believe that there was anything in that box. I spoke to the bereaved parents and later visited them. This was difficult for us all because their memories of him were not mine. However, as I was the last person to see their son alive, my presence seemed to give them some comfort. The doctor gave me more tranquillizers and told me to forget. I got the same advice from the policeman to whom I had to give evidence for the inquest. Easier said than done. During all this I had asked to see the body, to no avail. When I first heard the news I offered to identify the body. My offer was ignored and his father had to make a long journey to do so. Later, at home before the funeral, I asked my father if I would be allowed to view the body and was given an emphatic no. To this day I don't know whether it was red tape or parental sensibility which denied me a last look at someone I had loved.

Had I been less shocked at the time I would have pursued matters more forcibly. One argument against it seemed to be that I would be upset to see the damages inflicted by the car crash. Of course it would have been upsetting, but it would also have served to convince me that no spark of life could have remained in the body. As it was imagination is often the worse thing to cope with than reality. I could only visualize the body as a still version of the boy I knew. Intellectually I knew he was dead: subconsciously I couldn't give him up.

Outwardly I recovered quickly. I threw myself into work and thereby gained my graduate year at Cambridge and there met a loving, patient man to whom I am now, 12 years later, happily married.

But for much of that time I was plagued by dreams or daydreams. I would imagine that a mistake had been made, that my boyfriend was unharmed, simply with a loss of memory and that we would meet again.

I strongly believe that had I been allowed to see the body these distressing dreams would have faded long before they did. The practice of 'lying-in' which gives people a chance to see the body is a highly sensible act of mercy. The people left behind realize that what goes on at the funeral contains no life essence of the person they knew. This leaves them free to mourn in the clear knowledge of death and to take comfort from the funeral and friends. To deny this to anyone is a great cruelty and simply lengthens the process of coming to terms with the death.

It was only a few years ago that my dreams stopped. That was in spite of three children and a husband I love. But I owe them better than that. Next time a loved one dies I shall make sure I see the body so that my grief does not linger too long.

(Reprinted with kind permission of Polly Bird, 1989)

THE TIME OF DEATH

The nurse's role is crucial here because she is usually the professional carer who is most closely involved and may have had the opportunity to build up a relationship with the family.

We need to provide as much privacy as we can at the time of death so that the family can remain with their loved one to say goodbye in their own time and in their own way. It may be necessary to telephone other family members or friends on their behalf. The opportunity to sit for a while afterwards with someone from the ward team is very comforting. This could be any caring person, but preferably one who knew them and the person who died.

We need to be aware of all who are able to help and to liaise with them, introducing them to the family as needed. Those caring for the family may be doctors, nurses, social workers, volunteers, chaplain and the funeral director, and will often extend to the community with neighbourhood schemes, church groups, self-help groups and bereavement services of various kinds. These may, when necessary, supplement the family's own support networks of relatives, friends and neighbours and, where no such networks exist, provide evidence of caring concern helping the individual to feel part of life again.

Practical advice about what needs to be done is also valued at this time. Relatives need to know the arrangements for collecting the patient's belongings. This is still felt by many to be distressing, because of the way in which items which are precious to the deceased person – photographs, watch, jewellery, clothing, handicrafts etc. – tend to be piled into an orange sack, binliner or polythene bag of some kind.

Where these are handed over also requires sensitivity. Many relatives have expressed to me the wish to collect these from the ward where they can thank the staff at the same time. This makes an appropriate ending for them and is sometimes seen as an achievement, a challenge to which they have risen. However, this can only be rewarding for them if someone on the ward is able to give them the time when they arrive, and this is not always easy in practice.

When the patient has died it is of course, in one sense, an ending. The end of that life, certainly, also the end of our nursing role and the end of our relationship with the patient and his family. For close relatives leaving the ward for the last time, or seeing the community or Macmillan sister leaving their home, it is both an end and a beginning.

Most nurses I have met demonstrate commitment and skill when caring for dying patients. It is logical that, whenever possible, this care should extend to the bereaved person(s). In the community and in specialist units it is often possible to provide continuity of support with the nurse most closely involved with the family being able to visit after the death. I have found that this is much appreciated by close relatives who feel that they have not been forgotten.

This chapter has focused on needs at the time of death and the possible relationship between the meeting of these needs and the adjustment to bereavement that will eventually be made. It has also highlighted the nurse as a member of a team of people caring for relatives as well as for the patient.

REFERENCES

Ainsworth-Smith, I. and Speck, P. (1982) *Letting Go*, 2nd ed. SPCK, London.
Aries, Phillip (1974) *Western Attitudes to Death: from the Middle Ages to Present*, Johns Hopkins University Press, Baltimore.
Bird, Polly (1986) The *Guardian*, 14 May.
Clegg, Frances (1988) Cremation, burial and memorials: the options and choices of bereaved people. *Bereavement Care*, Vol. 7 (2), Summer.
European Public Health Committee (1981) *Problems Related to Death: Care for the Dying*, Final Report. European Public Health Committee, Strasbourg.
Freihofer, P. and Felton, G. (1976) Nursing behaviours in bereavement: an explanatory study, *Nursing Research*, Vol. 25, pp. 332-7.
Gibran, Kahlil (1978) *The Prophet*, William Heinemann, London.
Hempel, Sandra (1988) No place to lose a loved one, *Nursing Times News Focus*, Vol. 84 (35), 31 August.
Longbottom, Paul (1986) *Bereavement: an opportunity for the Church*, unpublished research project.
Which? Guide (1986) *What to Do When Someone Dies*, Consumers' Association, London.
Wright, A., Cousins, J. and Upward, J. (1988) *Matters of Life and Death: A Study of Bereavement Support in NHS Hospitals In England*. Kings Fund Project Paper no. 77, London.

5. Prolonged or Complicated Mourning

Nothing becomes so offensive so quickly as grief. When fresh it finds someone to console it, but when it becomes chronic, it is ridiculed, and rightly.

Seneca (*c*. 5 BC–65 AD)

INTRODUCTION

So far we have looked at patterns of grieving which are considered to be 'normal', and I use this word in the sense of being the most frequently found sequence of reactions. These are often referred to as normal grief reactions or uncomplicated mourning. However, some people fail to grieve in the usual way or take much longer than average to reach a particular phase. Indeed, for a few people the goal of adjustment and acceptance will never be reached, and this can be hard for us and their families to accept.

Responses become unusual when they differ in severity or in duration. Indicators that things may go wrong include a complete lack of response to the death as if it has not been comprehended, a state of shock that lasts for weeks rather than days, the acute pain of grief that lasts for months rather than weeks and/or what appears to be an excessive amount of guilt or remorse. A frequently found example of this potential problem is when a bereaved person seems to be unable to let go of mourning, feeling as if any move to a new way of life or possible enjoyment of living is essentially an act of betrayal of the deceased person.

In order to provide effective assessment, knowledge of what is usual must be the starting point (Figure 5.1; Table 5.1). However, there is no one indicator or set of clues that alone means the bereaved person is at risk. The factors shown in Figure 5.1 and Table 5.1 should be borne in mind when referring a bereaved relative to the care of the primary health care team and/or bereavement support services (professional or voluntary).

CLUES THAT *MAY* INDICATE COMPLICATED GRIEVING

- Avoidance of the grieving process by whatever means – by sheer effort of will, or by prolonged use of tranquillizers or antidepressants; a delay in expressing feelings of grief for more than two weeks; avoidance of any death–related rituals, customs or activities.
- Extreme expressions of self-blame, including a need for atonement; self-desctructive impulses which often go together with low self-esteem.
- Identification and idealization problems, feeling that the person who died is everywhere and was perfect and that they are directing one's life. This is a form of denial where the individual cannot contemplate having an independent existence. There may be a compulsion to imitate the dead person. (Pincus (1976) suggests that one is internalizing, or taking over, the love object so that it is not lost.)
- A history that indicates unresolved grief (from a previous loss). Some apparently minor events trigger off an intense grief reaction. For example, a lady who was bereaved a year before ran over and killed a rabbit. Her shock and regret appeared at first to be very normal reactions, but she experienced intense grief reactions, particularly feelings of self-blame, which lasted for several weeks.
- Preserving the environment of the deceased just as it was when the death occurred thus creating a shrine. Regarding *every* belonging and association as sacred (after a year). This does *not* mean that keeping some clothes, mementoes or a special place is abnormal; many people keep a special corner of the house (or garden), often with a photograph.

Figure 5.1   The bereavement process – an approximate time scale

Before the death	Time of death	Six weeks	Nine months	Two years
Shock Denial Anticipating grief Isolation Anxiety Fear of the future	Shock Numbness Denial Yearning or withdrawal/ hysterical clinging behaviour	Anger, bitterness Blame Guilt Searching Lack of concentration Loneliness Indecision Physical symptoms (they may be similar to those of the person who died)	Sadness Depression Loss of status Feelings of being stigmatized Loneliness Aimlessness	Acceptance of reality Adjustment Recovery New patterns of living Personal growth Gradual hope

Table 5.1 Factors that may affect the outcome of bereavement

The bereaved person	Their relationship with the person who died Age Previous experiences of illness/loss/death Culture Perception of their loss: What do I feel? What *should* I feel? Their usual health problems Any chronic disease General practitioner support Primary health care team support (if needed)
Family/dependents	Children, their ages and health Parents, their ages and health Siblings, their ages and health In-laws, their ages and health
The death	Anticipated/unexpected Where it took place: home/hospital/old people's home/maternity unit etc. The way in which they died: could it have been prevented? Age of the person who died The will
Social factors	Primary support group – people known for over five years Networks: neighbours/friends/regular social contacts Responsibility: for others (including pets) Responsibility: work Housing Financial status Usual hobbies: belongs to clubs/classes/sports
Religion	Funeral arrangements Minister/church support Observance of accepted customs Previous belief system
Miscellaneous	Anniversaries Other reminders Previous and subsequent bereavements Other previous and subsequent losses New interests – work/hobbies etc. Use of resources and services available

- A hypochondriacal fear of the illness from which the dead person suffered. This may not surface until an anniversary or when an individual reaches the same age. For example, a lady whose mother died of carcinoma of the colon suffered the same nausea and constipation; it was nearly two years before these physical symptoms subsided.
- A very radical and sudden change in lifestyle, especially if it excludes lifelong friends and usual activities. The substitution of another close relationship which is made very hastily, without grieving the loss of the previous one, such as marriage that takes place very soon after a death, or a sudden move to a new unknown part of the country.
- Depression as an illness, when unusually severe or prolonged. However, a total absence of depression *may* also be abnormal.

Other factors to bear in mind include: the sudden death of a spouse; isolation from family and other networks; a timid, clinging personality; an ambivalent relationship with the deceased; bad reactions to previous separations; cultural traditions that discourage the expression of emotion; the additional stress of severe financial problems or deep family rifts and quarrels, such as a post-bereavement family row.

Any one of these may be a clue that grieving is, or might become complicated. However, although they should concern us, any one may be appropriate for any individual at a particular time.

However, Parkes (1972) does point out that there is a better prognosis for recovery from pathological bereavement reactions than from most other forms of mental illness, which is very encouraging.

UNRESOLVED GRIEF REACTIONS

Hodgkinson (1980) suggests that people with unresolved grief reactions are generally referred to the psychiatric services, but not necessarily with grief as the presenting problem. He refers to a 1959 study of a group of 135 agoraphobics. The researcher, Roth, had found that 37 per cent had developed the problem soon after a bereavement or sudden illness in a close relative or friend.

He also quotes Ramsey (1976) who was one of the first to suggest a similarity between abnormal grief reactions and phobias. A phobia is described as consisting of anxiety towards and avoidance of an object or situation that is harmless. The avoidance prevents the individual from finding that the anxiety can diminish in the presence of the feared situation. Ramsey suggests that a bereavement is similar in being a single traumatic event leading to strong emotional reactions. Following the bereavement, objects, places etc. connected with the deceased produce strong reactions and so tend to be avoided if at all possible.

Thus the bereaved may become more distressed and depressed over time because it is known that when strong reactions are produced for short periods (when the bereaved are unable to avoid the reminders that produce the anxiety) they tend to increase, not decrease, in intensity. As well as being aware of the need to look for early signs of phobias, one must also look for signs of protracted depression and indications of addictive behaviour, particularly undue reliance on alcohol. Probably the best known example of chronic grief was Queen Victoria, who grieved for Prince Albert for the rest of her life.

AT RISK GROUPS

One problem we find if we are considering at risk groups (and this is so in any area of care) is that the majority of people could be perceived as falling within one. When brainstorming this question in workshops and other teaching situations, the list on the board keeps growing until we call an arbitrary halt!

Yet, some kind of categorization is needed if any kind of assessment and follow-up support is to be offered. I suggest that it is not only idealistic but unrealistic to aim for a support service of any kind (statutory or voluntary) for every bereaved person. I have argued earlier that this is superfluous for some people and that even if it seemed desirable on humanitarian grounds, it would be impossible to achieve. If you agree with me, then the next step must be to consider where the limited resources that are or could be available should be concentrated.

Parkes (1972) has classified five groups of people who may be more likely to react pathologically to bereavement and so might benefit from outside interventions of various kinds, and these provide a useful starting point.

Group 1: The image-conscious individual

You may be surprised to know that this title refers to you and me! We take on the professional role of nurse and in so doing become accustomed to being a helper in most situations. We are givers of care and help and, much less frequently, the recipients. Therefore there are two sides of this problem coin. We may well find it very difficult to ask for help from others or to accept it if it is offered to us. We may see this as meaning we cannot cope, and we tend to value coping very highly. On the other hand, it may also be hard for others to offer us support. They may think of us not as individuals but in terms of our role and have the expectation that we are able to accept and cope with any crisis in our lives. Parkes points out that prime examples from this group are general practitioners and ministers and their respective wives. I think the clergy do provide a thought-provoking example. Few of us might consider their need for understanding and support or even the possibility that their faith might even temporarily be shaken, for we expect them to provide us with answers and give us the confidence of their own certainty.

Group 2: The ambivalent relationship

All human relationships have at least an element of ambivalence in them. In this case we are concerned with those who had an unhappy relationship with the deceased. Contrary to what one might at first suppose, they are less likely to be able to adjust and this is linked to feelings of guilt and resentment. There are likely to be many regrets and more difficulty in coming to terms with any negative feelings. It may also be harder if there are fewer happy memories to recall when the initial preoccupation with the last period of the deceased's life has passed. Obviously there are particular problems where there were deep rifts or unresolved conflicts prior to the last illness or, worse still, before the death occurred. This can also happen in a previously stable relationship, prior to a sudden death, causing great anguish and regret to the bereaved person.

It can also grow gradually over a long period of ill-health, a common example being the deterioration of an elderly person, when a previously good relationship may be undermined by the demands of long-term care and the guilt that so often ensues from the caring of close relatives.

Group 3: The isolated individual

This refers to the person, often though not always elderly, who has little or no regular contact with family, friends or neighbours. They may always have been the kind of person who 'keeps themselves to themselves', or their way of life may have precluded much contact with others. The networks that most people tend to take for granted are absent, they are not known at particular shops, or by their milkman or postman, nor do they belong to community groups. A relevant example of this group is provided by the many couples who retire to the seaside or the country, leaving behind the networks of a lifetime, not realizing the security and starting point that these can provide in a crisis. Often one of the partners dies soon after this move and the bereaved person is left isolated. A comment I have had frequently made to me in this situation is 'We only lived for each other, we didn't need anyone else.' This sounds romantic when both partners are alive and well but is a devastating statement to make when one is finally alone.

People in this group need much practical help as well as encouragement, to venture out and make new contacts and friends. As they tend to have been non-joiners beforehand, or else they have only made contact with others as part of a pair, it is futile to suggest ways in which they could make new friends without taking account of the practical barriers. For example, if suggesting that a bereaved person attend a local meeting of Cruse (the Association for Widows and Widowers) it is usually necessary to introduce them to a member first so that they can be collected and attend with someone rather than make their own arrangements and go alone, no matter how warm the welcome when they actually arrive. It is also important to remember that for a few people their isolation is deliberately chosen. They may have a below-average need for human contact and well developed inner resources. However, it is not difficult in practice to determine the few individuals who do fall within this subgroup.

Group 4: The overdependent relationships

We have already seen that in any relationship we are to some extent dependent on the other person to reinforce our personality, to help us to know who or what we are. I am sure that you can think of a few people you know or have nursed at some time, where there appears to be an exaggeration of this and one person is very dominant and the other very subservient. Of course, each is in fact very dependent on the other and whichever one is bereaved they may feel excessively lost without the other. I tend to think of the two as constituting a pair of scales that become totally unbalanced when the weight on one side is removed. It can be hard for either to function at all without someone to dominate or be dominated by.

However, I can remember two examples of this kind of relationship where the dominant person was the one who died. My colleages and I considered the remaining half of a sister relationship, and the wife of a very dominant retired clergyman to be at risk, but in both cases the bereaved person emerged after their initial mourning stronger and more able to cope with all aspects of their lives than had seemed possible before. I can only speculate as to whether this would have been different if they had been the dominant ones. Perhaps you can think of one or two examples from your own experience that may underline or refute the hypothesis.

Group 5: Past history of emotional crisis

In this group are those who already have a history of being unable to cope adequately with stressful events in their lives. Losing someone close to you must be one of the most highly stressful life events any of us have to face so it is not difficult to see that previous difficulties with coping indicate a likelihood of problems with bereavement. A history of mental illness, particularly endogenous depression, may also be significant. In problems with adjustment there is frequently found a past bereavement or deep experience of loss which has never been fully explored or resolved by the individual. This points to the need, wherever possible, to discuss the background of the bereaved person, looking at previous ways they have resolved stressful events in their lives.

SUDDEN DEATH (AS OPPOSED TO ANTICIPATED DEATH)

Those whose loss was sudden and unexpected are, as one might suppose, more at risk of prolonged or complicated mourning. They have had no opportunity to grieve in advance of their loss. The death may have been from a road traffic or other accidents, or from sudden illness such as coronary artery disease or cerebrovascular accidents. Sudden deaths appear to be more difficult to grieve for than other kinds of death. They leave the survivor with a marked sense of unreality. Guilt feelings and an overwhelming need to direct anger at others and blame them for the death are particularly strong. Unfinished business is another definite concern with deep regrets for issues not discussed, love not expressed, or future decisions not shared with the deceased.

The overwhelming need many bereaved people feel strongly after a sudden death, is to see the body of the person who has died. This need was finally recognized after the Falklands war (in 1982) when the bereaved relatives were given the opportunity to visit the Falkland Islands and so be able to visualize the place where their loved ones died, and say 'goodbye' to them there, or else to have the body of their dead relative flown home to them.

Unexpected death often leaves many practical problems, particularly financial ones. These increase feelings of anxiety and insecurity and they may also delay the grieving process. A bereaved person with these kind of practical problems to resolve may have little or no time for anything other than survival. Though this may carry them through the first weeks or months, the sense of shock and early realization may well be delayed and have to be experienced much later. Family and friends may then misunderstand and not support the bereaved person who has apparently coped well for a long time and then appears to regress.

Sudden death, by its very nature, happens with little or no emotional preparation. Death may not have been discussed in the family at all. It may well be the bereaved person's first major loss and they have to face it without the person closest to them to support them.

A striking example of this need is provided by a lady I visited, in her mid-fifties; she had a grown up family and went out to work. Her husband was the head of a large language school. He had no previous history of any serious illness, nor even early symptoms of one, but one day they both went out to work as usual but he did not return. He had had a massive myocardial infarction while at a meeting that afternoon and died. His colleagues were unable to contact her until she was back at home in the evening, cooking supper.

For the next few weeks, she appeared to her family to be coping magnificently. She attended to all the practical details, appeared remote but dignified at the funeral and calmly outlined plans for the future. From time to time his colleagues and their friends asked her if there was anything they could do to help. After a while she summoned up the courage to tell them that what she wanted was for them to re-enact that meeting, as far as possible as they could, with her present so that she could make some kind of picture of it in her mind and 'believe in it'. We can only imagine how they must have felt at this request, but because she was a very forceful lady they eventually agreed. They described to her what happened and to some extent acted it out and she was aware that they felt very uncomfortable when she wanted to know the details such as in what direction he fell, who went over to him first, who telephoned the ambulance, etc. During this description, she suddenly broke down and wept. Immediately one of them turned to her and said, 'There, I told you we shouldn't have done this!' However, it was not until that moment that she believed he had really died and it was only then she could begin to mourn his loss.

This illustrates for us the importance of describing and explaining what happened to the bereaved person who was not present at the death, and encouraging them to feel comfortable about asking questions. This is probably needed by many bereaved people where the death was expected but they were either unable or unwilling to be present at the time.

The bereaved person also knows that the person who died had no time to grieve, to make plans, to express their wishes. They may feel that their most basic trust in life has been undermined by the death. There may also be certain aspects of the way in which the death occurred that make it harder to accept. An example is the 'double grief' which has been described as happening to the relatives of someone dying suddenly with myocardial infarction – they have lost the person, and also lost the value of that person having the chance to fight it. Early reactions to unexpected death may be misunderstood or mishandled.

It is often thought unwise to leave someone alone in case they 'do something silly', a euphemism for commiting suicide. If this is done clumsily the bereaved person may not want to be treated as if they are incapable, or to be overprotected.

The bereaved may need to ask questions again and again and express doubts and fears. For example, the whole truth may be withheld, the rationale given that it is to protect them. These withheld truths make what really happened appear not to make sense. The bereaved cannot understand and yet sense that they are being 'fobbed off', leading to further confusion and anxiety.

Having looked at the usual patterns of grieving (in Chapter 1) we have considered some of the factors that may make this process more complicated and protracted. We began by looking at some groups of people who *may* be more likely to have problems in bereavement. We concluded by looking at the particular problems of sudden (as opposed to anticipated) death.

In the next two chapters we shall look at other groups who have the potential to be 'at risk' during bereavement. However, in doing so we must be realistic about the limitations of such an approach. Not everyone who fits neatly into one of these categorizations will be 'at risk', neither can we assume that the others will *not* be.

REFERENCES

Hodgkinson, P. E. (1980) Treating abnormal grief in the bereaved, *Nursing Times*, 17 January.

Parkes, C. M. (1972) *Bereavement: Studies of Grief in Adult Life*, Tavistock, London.

Pincus, Lily (1976) *Death in the Family: The Importance of Mourning*, Faber and Faber, London.

Ramsey, R. (1976) A case study in bereavement therapy, in Eysenck, H. (ed) *Case Studies in Bereavement Therapy*, Routledge and Kegan Paul, London.

6. At Risk Groups: Death at the Beginning of Life – Death and Children

How can I teach, how can I save, this child whose features are my own.
Whose feet run down the ways where I have walked.

Michael Roberts (1902–48)

INTRODUCTION

The first part of this chapter considers the needs of families who lose a child either before or after birth. The second part considers the range of reactions and probable needs of children and adolescents who are bereaved, putting these in the context of at risk groups.

LOSING A CHILD BEFORE OR AFTER BIRTH

Infertility

The experience of not being able to have a child of one's own can be a devastating loss that can be likened to other kinds of 'hidden' bereavements, so called because they are often unrecognized by others. It can be a long series of losses as different treatments are tried and hopes are continually disappointed. 'Every period is a loss. It's like being bereaved every month,' said one colleague.

Miscarriage

The loss of a baby may take place so early that few family or friends even know that it has happened. In spite of this, it can cause much grief and mourning for the lost child, the extent depending on what the pregnancy meant to the parents. If the pregnancy was desperately wanted then the grief is likely to be acute and accompanied by feelings of failure. 'There is obviously something wrong with me,' explained a colleague who had lost a longed-for child at ten weeks gestation, 'because I can't do what all the other women I know can do. I am not "meant" to be a mother, I'm not good enough.' The notion that she was not in some way 'good enough' demonstrated a common feeling that the miscarriage is a kind of punishment, and is the individual's fault. A series of miscarriages can leave a woman obsessed with the need to have a child.

Abortion

Abortion can also give rise to grief reactions even when it has been decided upon with little inner conflict. Feelings of relief may still be accompanied by feelings of sadness and regret. However, often the decision has been made with great difficulty, to please others perhaps, or because of poor social and economic circumstances or because the mother has felt inadequate. Although abortion clinics in England are required to provide some kind of counselling service prior to the abortion, some girls I have spoken to expressed a fear of showing the slightest ambivalence about their decision, for fear that the abortion might be delayed or withheld altogether. The feelings of guilt and regret may be denied afterwards, especially as family and friends may expect the women to feel relieved and grateful for having the 'problem' solved. Therefore, this kind of bereavement may be unresolved, only to surface much later in a woman's life. For example, I remember a young girl of 22 who had advanced cancer, sharing with her medical social worker the anger and self-disgust she felt after having an abortion some years earlier. She did not want the social worker to tell the consultant, in case this lowered his opinion of her and, she felt, might even withdraw his care. This shows the extent of the guilt and low self-esteem the abortion had caused her, a burden that she carried with her until she was able to express it before she died.

Abortion after amniocentesis

Abortion performed because of genetic abnormality found after an amniocentesis test is clearly particularly distressing for the parents and family. The knowledge that the fetus was abnormal is likely to cause the same feelings as in loss of a healthy child which is experienced by parents whose baby is found to be handicapped at birth. Although mothers are asked before this test if they are willing to have a termination if the fetus is found to be abnormal, it is difficult if not impossible to be able to anticipate what their feelings may be.

The test cannot be performed before the sixteenth week of pregnancy and the results may take up to four weeks to be processed. In the meantime, the mother will experience the first movements of the fetus inside her; this makes the baby even more real to her and so increases feelings of attachment. She then has to have complete faith in her doctors, to accept the unpalatable truth they offer her that the baby who is now so real to her, its movements indicating health and viability, should be deliberately killed by her because it does not conform to the norms of this society. An example of the extreme grief and conflict was provided for me by the daughter of an elderly lady I nursed at home at one time. This daughter had married in her late thirties and had produced a healthy baby girl. She and her husband were keen that this should not be an only child, and soon after she became pregnant again at the age of 41. Her health was good and when she was offered an amniocentesis test she nearly did not accept it: 'I didn't really think it was necessary, having had one healthy child already. I didn't seriously think that the baby I was carrying could possibly be abnormal.' However, her husband thought it was a good idea and so she went ahead with it. Her shock on hearing the results two weeks later was profound. She remembers little of the decision to have a termination, 'I was just swept along, it didn't seem real.' But afterwards her anger and self-blame were acute.

> It was *my* baby, and I killed it. I committed murder. They say he would have been very handicapped, but how can they know how bad he would have been? There is so much that can be done now. I loved him, he was mine, and I allowed them to take him away from me. I deserve anything that happens to me now.

With professional help and a supportive family this lady was eventually able to come to terms with what happened.

The importance of recognizing the profoundly traumatic effect on women of the late termination of an often desperately wanted pregnancy cannot be overemphasized. The opportunity to talk about this wound to themselves and their relationship can be healing. A lady quoted in the *Sunday Times* (Dunn, 1985) said, 'Before, it was as if we had to shut it up in some Victorian chapel. I blamed myself for this gene. Now I don't. It's all out in the open, its part of our lives and we're coming to terms with it.'

The adoption of the new chorion villus sampling test that can be done as early as eight weeks of pregnancy may do much to alleviate this problem, although it carries a higher risk of miscarriage. The potential distress of early abortion or miscarriage still exists and it does not seem likely that it can provide an easy solution for any woman in the position of having to choose whether or not to terminate her pregnancy because of handicap.

Stillbirth

Stillbirth can happen quite unexpectedly or with little warning. It comes at the end of the pregnancy when usually the mother, and often the father as well, have begun to become attached to the forthcoming baby. It is particularly traumatic for the parents when it is known beforehand that the baby has died and the mother still has to face the process of labour but with no baby at the end of it. It is sometimes suggested that the process of labour may still be therapeutic, but it is difficult to understand why.

It must also be remembered that stillbirth raises particular stress for the midwives and doctors concerned. Not only does death at the time of birth turn over the natural and usual pattern of events, but it may also be that the bereaved parents, in their anger, attach some blame either overtly or via more subtle suggestion to midwifery or medical staff who were in charge at the time.

The Kohner Report on Midwives and Stillbirth (1984) focused on the midwives themselves, both in their professional role and as people, identifying the need to allow the midwife the freedom to be herself in this situation while at the same time acting professionally.

It is now recognized that many parents have a need to be able to hold and touch their stillborn baby. In the past, the usual policy was to remove the baby as quickly as possible, which could leave parents with a sense of unreality. Fantasies about what the baby looked like could be far worse than the truth. As we see in other situations, it helps the mourning process to know who it is one is grieving for and to be able to picture what actually happened.

Most help is directed towards the mother, but the needs of the father also have to be borne in mind. It is likely to help the future relationship of the parents if the experience can be shared.

An excellent booklet called *A Little Lifetime* (published by the Irish Health Education Bureau and SANDS) aimed at the parents of a stillborn baby or one who died shortly after birth, makes a very useful list of possible decisions for parents to consider making at that difficult time. These come under the headings of memories, keepsakes and naming your baby and would, I feel, be worthwhile remembering by any health professionals who may be involved.

The section on 'memories' makes the important point that parents who have not wanted or felt able to see their baby initially have every right to change their minds later and ask for it to be arranged then. If the death was not expected, the shock may be so great that they are unable to decide what they want. Other family members, particularly other children, may also want to see and hold the baby and it is helpful to give them the chance. If the parents prefer not to do so then they should be supported in that decision. The staff involved should feel able to offer to discuss and describe the baby and what happened when and if the parents wish it. All these suggestions are designed, of course, to help the parents accept their loss, the first task being to accept the reality of it, as with other kinds of bereavement.

'Keepsakes' is about other kinds of reminders that the baby was real, so that the parents have a focus for their grief. Staff involved can tactfully offer other mementoes such as the baby's identification bracelet, information about his weight, height and any other measurements; a lock of hair can be kept.

Depending on the maternity unit involved, it may be possible to supply a hospital certificate of the birth, also a baptismal certificate if the baby was baptised. A photograph is, of course, the ultimate reminder and most hospitals now take one that can be kept in the notes and given to the parents at any time they wish.

'Naming your baby' stresses the importance of giving the baby a name so that it can be used when discussing the baby with others, particularly children in the family. Again, it helps to make the baby real to them as well as to the parents. It also emphasizes the important point that this name should not be passed on to any subsequent children. This refers to potential problems to later children who may be conceived and brought up as substitutes or replicas of how the parents·imagine the dead baby would have been. There is always a danger that bereaved people will idealize the person who died and this can be especially difficult if this was a dead baby and later children are not seen as separate beings but as a kind of second best, living in place of the baby who died.

This booklet also points out to parents the importance of coming to a decision about some kind of burial or funeral service for the baby. It has been suggested that if some kind of funeral service is not performed, then parents come to regret this later. An example of this was shown on the Esther Rantzen BBC programme 'The Lost Babies' where one lady had grieved for 30 years because she did not know where her baby was buried nor had been given the chance to say goodbye.

Midwives and others involved in discussing these matters with the parents should be able to ensure that they have been consulted about any other aspects that are related to a final ritual of some kind. For example, the parents may wish the baby to be dressed in a particular outfit or be wrapped in a special shawl. There may be a particular toy or family memento that they would like to have placed by the baby. They may want to put a birth and/or death notice in the newspaper. Where there has been a close relationship with the midwife, it is not unusual for the parents to want them to be present at any ceremony decided upon.

Because stillbirth is still, in most senses, a 'hidden' loss parents may feel distress when others appear to forget the baby or expect them to have adjusted to the loss very quickly. On anniversaries and special occasions they may need to remind other family members that their baby existed and that his loss is still mourned.

Neonatal death

The environment of the special care baby unit is an alien one and its impact on the family is likely to be powerful. As Vas Dias (1987) writes so eloquently ' . . . there are masses of complicated clicking, buzzing, whirring, ringing machines and everywhere is a sense of walking a tightrope while attempting to do something natural; take care of a newborn baby.'

Where the death is of a neonate, parents will grieve as for a stillbirth except that they, and often other members of the family such as grandparents and other children, will have got to know the baby even if only for a very short time. Therefore, the parents are mourning someone they knew, that they can picture permanently in their minds and whom they have usually had the opportunity to touch and hold. This means that they have begun the process of attachment to the baby and, in most neonatal units, will have been encouraged to be actively involved in its care. They are very likely to want to hold and cuddle the baby, although this can be difficult to achieve satisfactorily if the baby is in the intensive care unit. Nursing staff can help by giving them confidence and encouragement and involving them as much as possible. This is very important – they must not feel that their baby 'belonged' to the experts, making them feel inadequate and vulnerable.

Another area of potential difficulty is when there has been more than one birth and not all survive, for example where there have been twins and only one lives. The parents may well feel confused and torn between their feelings of sadness over the one who has died and the pleasure of the one who lives. Casual remarks such as 'At least you have one baby to bring home, which is more than some mothers have!' reported by one mother, can cause great unhappiness, implying that one baby is in some way interchangeable with another.

Such remarks are often reported to have been made by family or friends to bereaved parents and sometimes even by nursing and other professional staff. Any comments of the 'You can always have another one!' variety are particularly hurtful for this reason. It has to be remembered that the loss is not of the neonate but also of all the potential he had – it is the loss of a baby, a toddler, a school child, student or adult. A certain amount of anticipatory grieving is likely to be done by most parents of babies in special care units. The very fact that they are there means there is a sense of loss of the expected outcome of the pregnancy, and an awareness of the fragility and vulnerability of their baby. The accompanying anxiety and fears for the baby's future, including whether or not it is likely to grow and live normally afterwards, are likely to continue for some time after the baby is able to go home with them.

A practical problem following both a stillbirth and the death of a neonate, which can cause great discomfort and distress, is the continued production of breast milk. This hurts both physically and psychologically, the mother experiencing an intense sensation of needing to feed the baby. Medication can be very effective in relieving the physical symptoms of engorgement and should be offered to the mother.

Sudden infant death

One baby in every 500 live births dies unexpectedly for no obvious reason between the ages of one week and two years, 90% before eight months.

Although such tragedies are comparatively rare, in a group practice of two or three doctors a cot death is likely to occur every two to four years. A general practitioner may be called to the home or the baby rushed to the surgery; often the baby is taken direct to a hospital casualty department.

General practitioners should ensure in advance that coroners, hospital and medical deputizing services will inform him or her immediately of an unexpected infant death.

'Cot death' is the well-known term used to describe the sudden infant death syndrome (SIDS), which is the commonest cause of death in the early months of life and where no clearcut cause of death can be found. Each day in the United Kingdom, five babies die suddenly, silently and unexpectedly for no obvious reason, and it is this latter word that makes it particularly hard to come to terms with.

The Foundation for the Study of Infant Deaths has produced a very useful checklist aimed at helping doctors who are managing cot death for the first time, also nurses and health visitors; it is reproduced as follows, with kind permission of the Foundation for the Study of Infant Deaths (Cot Death Research and Support):

Checklist

The following notes were written to help doctors manage a cot death for the first time. I know several nursing colleagues in the community who have also found these to be helpful.

(1) As soon as you hear of the baby's death *contact the family* to express sympathy, by a home visit if possible. Early support prevents later misunderstandings.

(2) Unless there is obvious injury, a history of illness or the parental attitude arouses suspicion, tell the parents it appears to be a cot death but that a *postmortem* examination will be necessary to establish the cause of death. If death remains unexplained, it may be registered as sudden infant death syndrome. Some parents want to see or hold their child after death is confirmed but before the body is taken to a mortuary.

(3) Explain the *coroner's duty*, the possibility of an inquest, and warn parents that they or relatives may be asked to identify the body. Advise the parents that they will be asked to make a statement to the coroner's officer or police, and that bedding may be taken for examination to help establish the cause of death. If necessary, give advice on registering the death and making funeral arrangements.

Coroner's officer may need to know parents' choice of burial or cremation.

(4) If considering offering parents a drug to alleviate the initial shock, it is known that many do not want anxiolytics or antidepressants, but prefer something to *induce sleep*.

(5) If the mother was *breastfeeding*, give advice on suppression of lactation; prescribe medication and advise her to leave the breasts alone except to empty them once a day if an easy method is available.

(6) Take particular note of *siblings*. Remember that twin babies carry an extra risk of cot death and that a surviving twin may need hospitalization for observation. Give guidance on emotional needs of siblings, who may be neglected or overprotected; reassure parents that older children are not at risk.

(7) Advise parents of likely *grief reactions* such as aching arms, hearing the baby cry, distressing dreams, and strong positive or negative sexual feelings, but reassure them that these and other symptoms such as loss of appetite and sleeplessness are normal and temporary. Anger, sometimes directed towards the general practitioner, guilt and self-blame, especially on the part of the mother, are common grief reactions for which the doctor should be prepared.

(8) Offer parents copies of the leaflet *Information for the parents following the sudden and unexpected death of their baby* and the address of the *Foundation for the Study of Infant Deaths*. In addition to sponsoring medical research, the Foundation offers further support and information, and can put parents in touch with others who have previously suffered a similar bereavement.

(9) Make sure that parents have a *relative or close friend* very near them during the 48 hours after the death, and offer explanation to them and to the minister of religion. Make sure the family's health visitor and other members of the primary care team know of the baby's death and are prepared to give continued support.

(10) Arrange a subsequent meeting with the parents to *discuss the cause of death*. Make sure the coroner informs you of the initial and final postmortem findings and consult with the pathologist if any clarification is needed.

(11) Offer parents a *later interview with a paediatrician* both for themselves and the siblings. An independent opinion is mutually beneficial to the parents and general practitioner, restoring parental confidence in the primary care team and sharing some of the load of counselling concerning future children.

(12) Parents who have lost a baby unexpectedly will need extra attention and support with their *subsequent children* from their obstetrician, paediatrician, general practitioner and health visitor.

In this situation the parents and other family members have had ample time to be attached to the baby and the mother is intensively involved in caring from him. The whole pattern of her life will revolve around the baby, and indeed the whole household will be geared to attending to the baby's needs at this stage.

The suddenness and unpredictability of this death makes it particularly shocking both to the family and to friends and acquaintances in the community. 'Cot death' is fortunately rare enough for few people to have come across it before, but this means that it is totally outside their experience and is all the more dramatic and frightening because of the need for police involvement and questioning of the parents by them and by medical and social work personnel. Parental feelings of guilt are enhanced and they may feel that everyone around them is accusing them of neglect and violence towards their baby.

The majority of cot death victims are taken to the accident and emergency departments where it is usually obvious that the baby is dead. However, both the parents and the staff are likely to feel a great need to attempt to save the baby's life and to be seen to try to do so against all the evidence that is too late.

The parents will feel anxious to convince the staff that they did love and care for the baby and they may be very defensive when asked questions about the baby's state of health. Husbands and wives or other family members may, in their anger and their need to find a reason for the death, criticize and accuse each other, the need to blame being exacerbated by police involvement.

Not only should the opportunity be provided for the mother and father to hold the baby, but also for other close members of the family who wish it.

After a stillbirth, neonatal or cot death an important issue becomes whether to have another baby or not. As one mother put it, 'I feel I don't want another baby. I want the one who died!' Others feel they do want to try for another, while knowing it will never replace the one who died. Most will want guidance as to the feasibility of doing so.

The death of a child

The relationship between an adult and his or her children is a very special one and differs greatly from other kinds of relationships. It begins long before the actual birth, when it is physically part of its mother, living within her from the moment its existence is acknowledged, and some kind of relationship begins with both parents. Attachment to the future baby has started. Many pregnancies are unplanned and unwanted, either initially or throughout, and then the attachment is an ambivalent one but it still exists.

The death of one's child is always an untimely one, whether it takes place after a few weeks of life as a fetus or if it happens in adulthood, but before the death of the parents. In western society the universal expectation is that children do not die and this causes parents to feel guilty for their child's death, reflecting a fear that society will blame them for it.

It is often said to parents who have lost a child that, if there are other children, they will be a great comfort. In some ways this is true but they may not be at all times. Parents may easily lose their temper with other children and even feel resentful that they are alive and healthy. These feelings may cause guilt and self-reproach. Children who are, themselves, bereaved may be cruel and hurtful and parents may feel they never loved the brother or sister who died. Problems occur when parents look to the children for their own emotional support.

Death by violence

The violent death of a child produces a bereavement response which is protracted and may well never be resolved. Where the violence accompanies a war it may, to some extent, be socially sanctioned although the death of an innocent child cannot be justified even in terms of standing for a cause. The death of a child in some kind of natural disaster also cannot be justified as serving any purpose. The need to blame someone for the death is particularly strong.

Where the death has been caused directly by another as in the violence of murder, the start of grieving is usually delayed. The child may have been missing for hours, days or even longer and when the body is found it becomes the property of the Crown and there can be no funeral until the coroner releases it.

The postmortem and inquest further delay the burial of the body, and if someone has been convicted of murder the trial will be an additional trauma that puts off mourning. Murder investigations and the legal process can be drawn out for a long time and leave the bereaved parents and family with a sense of being in limbo, unable to grieve or to move forward in any way.

Understandably, this kind of death is especially difficult for other people in the community to be involved in, to offer help, because it is a situation that people have no previous experience of and it is particularly shocking, shaking the very foundations of the individual's sense of security. It provides a good example of the need for self-help, being able to talk about what has happened with others who have been through similar experiences, as the most valuable way of adjusting to their loss.

BEREAVEMENT IN CHILDREN AND ADOLESCENTS

Children and adolescents are particularly at risk during bereavement. We are aware that many people feel uncomfortable when attempting to communicate with bereaved people and, indeed, that they may try to avoid them altogether. These feelings of discomfort may be even more marked when meeting children who have been bereaved. This may be because children tend to be more direct, they may ask difficult questions and they may behave in seemingly inappropriate and unpredictable ways that can be hard to understand, especially by other family members who are also suffering reactions to bereavement.

Concept of death

Even an infant appears to be able to sense the emotionally charged atmosphere of a griefstricken family, and to react to the absence of someone to whom he has become attached. Bowlby (1980) suggests that even as early as the last part of their first year, infants are able to hold in their heads the concept of a person and, therefore, to look for them when they are not present. Bowlby describes the death of the prime attachment figure (usually, of course, the mother) as causing the experience of separation even in an infant, and this is composed of the strong emotions of protest, then despair and then detachment, the latter leading to withdrawal behaviour or distracting activity which can be intense and aggressive.

Lansdown (1985) points out that the concept of death is one which evolves gradually, between six or seven years of age. She goes on to point out that it is often argued that a child's own experiences will affect the development of the concept. It is predictable that children who have themselves experienced the death of a relative, close friend or a pet, would have an accelerated concept. She also quotes a study by McWhirter (1980) of children in Northern Ireland. When living in one of the areas of violence, they did demonstrate a more advanced definition of death even as early as four or five years.

It would appear, therefore, that up to approximately school age loss through either death or absence has a similar effect. Between five and eight years children are still very egocentric and, while having more understanding of the concept, they tend to believe that a death is in some way their fault, so they feel guilty as if it is a punishment for misbehaviour. At this stage they may still think that is reversible. Like adults their reactions will depend on personality and previous ways of coping, as well as on their age. One eight-year-old went into school and straightaway told his best friend and teacher about the death of his grandmother. His twin brother never mentioned this to anyone at school either that day or afterwards.

Death of a parent

Black (1986) makes the important point that children can only mourn something that is actually within their experience of life. She cites an example of a nine-year-old girl who only five hours after the death of her father asked, 'Will Mummy get married again?' She was asked why she wanted to know and replied, 'Because if she did we would have to move house.' Black explains that this girl has been without her father for only five hours which was a usual experience and so 'all right'. She had previously moved house and lost her friends and had not liked that experience at all. Therefore, she was mourning what she knew. It is not hard to imagine how easily this could have been misunderstood by others and cause great distress.

A child who has lost a parent may be secretly afraid of losing the other one so explanation and information is important at any age, particularly as children tend to fill in the gaps in their knowledge with fantasies. What they imagine may well be more harmful to them than the truth, and those of you who have nursed children may have found that they accept painful realities more readily than do many adults.

It is often changes in behaviour that indicate to us if a child is not able to adjust to bereavement. Even adolescents cannot always be expected to put painful feelings and strong emotions into words (and neither, for this matter, can many adults!). A troubled child often regresses to an earlier stage of development and may start, for example, to wet the bed again, or bite their nails or have nightmares. The extrovert child who usually likes the company of many friends may withdraw and want to be alone, the shy, quiet child may become loud and aggressive.

It is usually the person closest to the child who is most deeply affected by the loss. They may be unable to offer the child all the attention and concern they need all the time. It may be helpful for someone outside the family, or not too deeply involved, to take a particular interest in the bereaved child for some time afterwards. They may help the child to make sense of what has happened and to understand the reactions of the other members of the family who may be upset and irritable. The re-assurance of someone well-known to them, who is able to be patient and loving can be very valuable in supporting them in their home situation.

Providing opportunities to talk about what has happened is also valuable but adults need to understand that children usually do not want long or complicated discussions. They may ask a question about the death, listen to the answer and then turn to a seemingly trivial and un-connected event. 'Has Mummy gone to heaven?' asked one seven-year-old, and in the next breath 'I'm building a Lego train!'

Professor Amartya Sen, speaking at the International Conference on Grief and Bereavement in 1988, expressed a concern which other parents whose partner has died have considered. While understanding the importance of talking openly with his children about his wife (who had died) he wondered how far he should go in initiating such discussion or whether he should leave this entirely to them. As time passes the question becomes more crucial. There is not, of course, an easy answer but it may be simplest to be guided by one's own feelings at the time, and aim for naturalness.

It is probably helpful to bear in mind that if the parent is obviously and frequently deeply upset by the mention of the dead parent, the children may become afraid to do so. The remaining parent represents, among other things, their security. It can be frightening and painful to witness great distress and they are likely to avoid doing so.

Death of a sibling

The death of a brother or sister adds a further dimension to these reactions. The grief felt is often compounded by strong feelings of guilt at the death of a rival. Their darkest wishes have been realized and so grief is mixed with strong feelings of both triumph and disaster. Children are very egocentric (as are some adults!) so they often have intense feelings of being responsible in some way for the death, which they may find hard to share with others.

Adolescents

The teenage years of childhood have the reputation of being turbulent ones. There are many developmental changes, both physically and mentally, and the new sense of power that this brings often, though not always, causes conflict within the family. Indeed, Lake (1984) makes the point that the finest achievement of parenthood in the animal kingdom is the attainment of full independence by the young of the species, yet for *Homo sapiens* the opposite seems very often to be true! Parents tend to discourage independent thought and action and to question any decision the teenager wishes to make, with the likely outcome, as Lake suggests, that the teenager stops reporting them honestly. This is, of course, only one facet of the potentiality for conflict between the teenager and his family. It is not hard to envisage the stresses that a bereavement could cause on a family unit, when superimposed upon an existing battleground.

It has even been suggested that teenagers go through a kind of mourning process as part of *normal* adolescence. This is composed of recognizing the loss of an idealized image of parents, the loss of one's own childhood, the loss of dependencies within the family and the loss of some unrealistic hopes and dreams for the future. This process leads to expressions of grief with expressions of anxiety and helplessness and the anger that often accompanies feelings of vulnerability. There is also a high likelihood of loneliness. These unhappy feelings are often not recognized or deliberately disregarded by adults such as the family, teachers and health professionals. Once again it can be seen that if the grief of bereavement is added to this existing distress the teenager may indeed be at risk of future emotional problems.

The death of a parent is likely to be the greatest loss at this time, especially if there has been a recent history of discord. The loss of a grandparent tends to be the first significant death a teenager faces and much will, of course, depend on whether this was a distant or close relationship. The loss may be a very significant one, and yet other adults may not realize its impact. The loss of an older brother or sister may represent the loss of a support and initiator into adult life, while the death of a younger one may be like losing a teenager's own baby or child.

The teenage years are noted for being a time when intense and intimate relationships are made with peers outside the family group. If the death of such a friend does occur, the remaining ones who valued them are likely to be deeply affected, yet they are often not recognized as being bereaved, least of all by the dead person's family. Grief may then be stifled and unexpressed leading to many potential future problems.

Goldacre (1987), a teacher and educational therapist, describes working at an inner city school in London where one of the teenage boys had been electrocuted on the local railway line. Many of the boys wanted to talk with her about the accident and, when the inquest was over, they told her the funeral was to be that afternoon. The deputy head, year master and tutor were going to represent the school. The boys asked if they could go too. Some teachers expressed doubts about this but eventually agreement was reached and they went. They had many practical questions to ask concerning the layout of the chapel and they wanted to go to the graveside afterwards. Many of the teachers thought this was inappropriate but the clergyman said they could do so if they wished. They stood together while other vehicles left, including the one carrying the dead boy's mother. She caught sight of them and recognized her son's best friend, and Goldacre says it was like 'the sun breaking through the clouds, though it was still raining, when she stopped weeping, smiled, waved and blew him a kiss.'

Back at the school the boys asked if she would talk to someone who had had a fight with the boy shortly before he was electrocuted because he was feeling very bad about it. She points out that their feelings had been looked after and so they were able, in turn, to look after someone else's.

There was some uncertainty as to why some of the boys had wanted to attend the funeral although Goldacre noted that at least one had recently lost his own mother. The teachers involved had come round to agreeing about the psychological value of the shared experience and also the comfort which the sight of them had brought the dead boy's mother. They had been helped to express and share grief which might well help to minimize behaviour problems later on.

Another less obvious loss that may be encountered in the teenage years is the loss through abortion, miscarriage or adoption of a girl's first pregnancy. Even though the girl may have agreed to relinquish the baby or the pregnancy and may appear to share society's view that it was a problem which has now been solved, she is likely to grieve for it. The boy who fathered it may also experience grief and will be even less likely to receive any understanding or support from adults.

There appears to be little conclusive evidence of long-term morbidity or premature mortality associated with bereavement in childhood and in the teenage years, nor any agreement about children of any particular age being more at risk after losing a parent. However, it appears likely that inhibited losses – those that are not explained or shared emotionally – may well contribute to vulnerability in adulthood, particularly to depression and possibly to suicide. Acknowledgement that the child has needs, coupled with sensitive support and security will, as with adults who are bereaved, help them to develop, to adapt and so to survive.

Adolescents tend to demonstrate a kind of pseudoadult behaviour as if trying to be grown up in order to master their insecurity. This may show in an almost compulsive desire to care for others in the family which may be construed by younger brothers and sisters as being bossy. If extreme, this can alienate others and make them think that the child is coping much better than they are. A bereaved lady I visited described the behaviour of her only daughter, aged thirteen, who since the death of her father had not left her alone. From when she made tea and had it in bed with her mother in the morning, to when she came downstairs to make her a night–time drink she was always with her. This lady expressed much guilt for feeling irritated at being fussed over and also anger at what she took to be a cold and even callous disregard for her need to be alone. She had begun to expect the girl of thirteen years to have the insight and understanding of an adult; she also felt that her daughter's behaviour meant that she did not need to grieve for her father. She did not think of the child's constant presence as to do with *her* need for security and fears that her mother might leave her too. Bowlby (1980) lists the factors that he believes will influence the outcome of a major childhood bereavement:

- The cause and the circumstances surrounding the death; this will include the information and explanation given to the child at the time and also subsequent answers to his questions and concerns.
- The quality of the relationship with the remaining family, especially with the surviving parent.

● The previous pattern of relationships within the family prior to the loss, especially between the parents and between the parents and that particular child.

Foster (1981) underlines the need for many caring adults, including health professionals and teachers, to be involved in helping the bereaved child and to encourage him to express his thoughts and feelings, so refusing to collude with denial. Offering explanations to children when no certain answers can be given should also be avoided. As with adults, honesty is more helpful in the longer term.

Attendance at the funeral

An issue that causes much debate and concern to adults is whether or not a particular child should attend the funeral of the loved person. There is no easy answer to this and it is necessary to explore the feelings of the child as far as this is possible. It would obviously not be helpful to force a child to do so, but it would seem that many children could benefit from having the opportunity if they were given the explanation and support. Once again, what they may imagine happens may well be more distressing than the reality. They are old enough to attend if they are able to sit through what is usually a very short service. If they choose not to go then they need the care of someone familiar while the family is away and to be able to discuss what happened afterwards as they feel the need. They may also need to visit the grave or go to the crematorium at a later date when it can be made a less stressed atmosphere with time to talk.

Those that choose to go need to have someone with them who is not too overcome by the loss and so is able to support them. They need to understand that the tears and signs of distress they see are because the loved one will be missed and not because something awful happens to the dead person after the funeral or when they die, and that this is a natural reaction.

In this chapter we have concentrated on the problems that can happen when death takes place at the beginning of life. We have discussed the concept of death in children and their possible reactions to loss within their family and friends, and the special needs of adolescents, an often neglected group.

REFERENCES

Ballard, Rod (1976) Sharing the pain – help for parents with a handicapped child. *Health Visitor*, Vol. 79, pp. 395–6.

Ballard, Rod (1982) Taking the family into account. *Mental Handicap*, Vol. 10 (3), pp. 75–6.

Black, Dora (1986) Bereaved children – family intervention. *Bereavement Care*, Vol. 2 (2).

Bowlby, John (1980) *Loss, Sadness and Depression*, Hogarth Press, London.

Dunn, Elisabeth (1985) Death before life. *Sunday Times*, 8 December.

Foster, Susan (1981) Explaining death to children. *British Medical Journal*, 14 February, pp. 540–2.

Foster, S. and Smith, P. (1987) 'Brief Lives', Thames TV series.

Goldacre, Patricia (1987) Working with bereaved boys in a secondary school. *Bereavement Care*, Vol. 6(2).

Health Education Bureau and Stillbirth and Neonatal Death Society (SANDS) (1986) *A Little Lifetime*. A booklet for parents whose babies have died around the time of birth. Health Education Bureau and the Stillbirth and Neonatal Death Society, Ireland.

Hill, Susan (1989) *Family*, Michael Joseph, London.

Kohner, Nancy (1984) *Report on Midwives and Stillbirth*. The Report of a Joint Royal College of Midwives/Health Education Council Workshop, October.

Kubler-Ross, Elisabeth (1983) *On Children and Death*, Macmillan, London.

Lake, Tony (1984) *Living with Grief*, Sheldon Press, London.

Lansdown, R. (1985) The development of the concept of death in childhood. *Bereavement Care*, Vol. 4(2).

McWhirter, L. (1980) Awareness of death in Belfast children. Paper presented at the Annual Conference of the British Psychological Society.

Oakley, Ann (1984) *Miscarriage*, Fontana, London.

Redshaw, M. E., Rivers, R. P. A. and Rosenblutt, D. B. (1985) *Born Too Early*, Oxford University Press, Oxford (particularly Chapter 5).

Sen, Amastya (1988) Children's and family grief and bereavement. Lecture given at the International Conference on Grief and Bereavement in Contemporary Society, Queen Elizabeth Conference Centre London, 14 July.

Vas Dias, Susan (1987) Psychotherapy in special care baby units. *Nursing Times*, Vol. 83(23), pp. 50–2, 10 June.

7. At Risk Groups: Death in Adulthood

The world breaks everyone, and afterwards many are strong in the broken places.

Ernest Hemingway (1899–1961)

INTRODUCTION

This chapter looks at bereaved adults who may be at risk. Possible problems related to the age, type and/or circumstances associated with the death will be considered in turn. The special problems that may be caused in the case of death by suicide are considered first.

SUICIDE

It is estimated that every day in England and Wales, eleven people take their own lives. According to Stengel (1969) a suicide act is 'any deliberate act of self-damage which the person committing the act could not be sure to survive'. It can also be argued that many forms of chronic behaviour are methods of indirect self-destruction, and could be viewed in a similar light.

It is often put forward that many suicide gestures are not intended to end with death, but are designed to draw attention to the individual and his problems. However, if a person gives even a hint of a specific plan to commit suicide, this should never be ignored. It has been suggested that contrary to the popular view, most suicidal people do, in fact, give advance warning of their intentions. They may give away precious possessions, make a will or make specific comments that indicate their intentions. Another sign to be aware of is the person who has been previously very distressed and who then becomes suddenly cheerful. This could mean that they have now decided on suicide as a solution to their problems.

Elderly people have higher suicide rates than those at other life stages, but they make fewer suicide attempts, tending to communicate their intentions to commit suicide less frequently and, therefore, being more successful (Moore, 1986).

This kind of sudden death linked to mental illness is one where the bereaved are likely to be particularly at risk. In this situation it is most likely that family, friends and neighbours will feel so uncomfortable that they are unable to offer support or to talk about what happened in any way and this increases the isolation of the bereaved person. The guilt they feel is more intense as they search for an explanation as to what their loved one actually meant by choosing to die.

Pete Murray (1983) writing in *The Times* about the suicide two years previously of his son Michael, says that

> The very hardest thing for me has been not to blame myself for what happened. Of course, I've tortured myself by wondering where I went wrong, and asking myself whether his death could have been prevented by more vigilance, better treatment (he suffered from bouts of depression), but that line of thinking just drags you and everyone else down, and achieves nothing.

Lake (1984) makes the distinction between two kinds of suicide, one a state of anger, the other an expression of fear. Anger suicide describes the violent statement that suicide makes about how the individual values his own body and the life it contains. This emotion is one the person has been unable to communicate fully or satisfactorily to those who matter to him. Frustration is suppressed anger, and suicide can be viewed as a last resort when the anger has been suppressed for so long that there is only one way left to show everyone the truth about the anger that has always been there.

Fear suicide indicates an extreme form of retreat from life. The fear of being alive becomes greater than the fear of death. Life is perceived as being hopeless and full of distress and pain and the individual no longer feels they have the strength to contend with the negativity of everything they see around them. The statement implied in this kind of death is likely to be one of sorrow rather than of anger. Sometimes it appears that the person wanted those left behind to feel as unhappy and lonely as they did, and perhaps through this to understand what they went through. Yet they are forcing those closest to them, as Lake suggests, to be anxious rather than angry, to miss somebody they did not love enough, rather than to be hurt by somebody whom they did not seem to love at all. It seems to say, you have forgotten me while I was alive and I challenge you by my death to go on forgetting me. Someone who has been close to, or tried to be close to, a person undergoing these feelings prior to suicide, is likely to have begun to feel the grief of bereavement before the death, even though they may not have recognized this at the time.

Probably one of the first and hardest tasks for someone bereaved by suicide is to accept the reality that their relationship with that person was not working well. They need to remember that this is true of many relationships between people, and that it does not usually lead to a suicide attempt. The dead person made the decision to make a dramatic statement about this and the bereaved person has every right to feel angry about that and to express this to others. They also need to work through feelings of guilt with the goal of accepting that each human being is ultimately responsible for themselves, therefore accepting or apportioning blame becomes irrelevant.

It may be useful for us to look at suicide in terms of it being the most drastic solution to the problem of grief. It represents the end of the pain of mourning with its attendant suffering, anguish and sense of isolation from others and from life itself. It may also be viewed as a way of being reunited with the person who died. The grieving person may decide that their remaining family would be better off without them. Hence the justification expressed by a young widow of small children, 'They'd be happier without me. I am always sad and irritable.'

In these terms it can be seen as being a rational thing to do when, as Oakley (1985) put it, 'the one real problem is life itself'. Parkes (1970) found from his studies that ideas of suicide were often expressed. Many of the London widows in his study went through a period during which they felt they 'might as well be dead' or 'if it wasn't for the children I might consider it'. However, he found only one widow in his sample who had made any sort of suicide attempt and that was described as being 'very half-hearted'.

Parkes and Weiss (1983) cite research that indicates that counselling the bereaved may reduce the incidence of suicide amongst them. They give as an example the bereavement counselling service which was introduced at St Christopher's Hospice in London, in 1984. In the six years preceding this, six bereaved relatives of patients who had died there were known to have committed suicide.

A wider perspective of the problem of suicide is provided by Stengel (1969) who reflected that 'social isolation is the common denominator of a number of factors correlated with a high suicide rate'. When discussing the possible prevention of it he comments that 'the fight against suicidal behaviour is only one of the aspects of a much bigger problem, which is the drastic reorganization of society to the social needs of its members'. This suggestion that, in a sense, we are all responsible for the suicide of an individual within our society – be they a bereaved person or someone with difficult relationships or with a stressful social situation – contrasts with the view of Lake (1984), already expressed, that ultimately no blame should be apportioned for the suicide of any individual, the last responsibility being entirely their own.

Stengel underlined the important factor of social isolation. For the bereaved person this is sometimes in part imagined, but it may also be uncomfortably true. The bereaved person's position may be threatening to others, reminding them of their own vulnerability. Margaret Torrie (1975) (the founder of Cruse and herself a widow) speaks of widowhood as 'entering the dark world of other people's fears'. The customary British reserve and horror of saying or doing 'the wrong thing' can mean that the bereaved person is actually avoided by others, and indeed many people have admitted to me during bereavement workshops that they have in the past deliberately avoided encounters with people they know have recently been bereaved. Reasons given for this have ranged from 'I was afraid that I might make them feel worse', 'I didn't know whether to mention the subject or not', or 'I didn't know what I would do if they cried', 'I could have just talked about the weather and things like that but it might have seemed as if I didn't care about what had happened'. In these examples one can see that there is a preoccupation with how the bereaved person would perceive them, rather than with the bereaved person's needs.

It appears feasible, therefore, that social isolation is a very real problem for many bereaved people, and if we accept that this may be an important factor in attempted and intended suicide it points to a need for us, as members of a community as well as nurses, to do what we can to change attitudes and help people towards more confidence in approaching the bereaved at whatever level of human contact may be appropriate for their relationship.

LOSS IN OLD AGE

The gradual process of ageing inevitably produces many types of loss. Green (1985) lists the main ones as being:

- loss of income;
- loss of bodily functions;
- loss of health;
- loss of independence, and house (including by admission to residential or nursing home or hospital);
- loss of sexual attraction;
- loss of company, for example spouse, friends, pets;
- loss of life.

Looking at this list one may be inclined to believe that the elderly are likely to make effective adjustments to bereavement, having learnt about the process of adjustment to other losses and having the expectation that the death of loved ones is an inevitable part of growing old. However, in practice this is not often found to be the case. Some of the elderly people I have visited have, in fact, the perception of much younger people and found it difficult if not impossible to accept that they themselves and their loved ones were, as was often put to me '*that* old' or 'we were getting on in years, but we were both very fit'. Many sons and daughters are not 'ready' for their parent to die. Yet people may expect them to feel little sorrow when an elderly parent dies.

Research into the reactions of bereavement has tended to be done on younger age-groups, and there seems to be a belief that the elderly suffer grief less than their younger counterparts and so the risk to their mental health is reduced. It is important to remember, when nursing elderly patients, that they may well have been recently bereaved, otherwise it is easy for their bereavement to go unacknowledged, and their feelings to be misunderstood.

However, there is some evidence to show that the high incidence of depression and of suicide in old age may be attributable to bereavement and that there is no justification for ignoring the problem. From one of his own studies (1964) Parkes concludes that elderly individuals were more vulnerable than younger ones to the physical effects of bereavement and that pre-existing chronic illness such as osteoarthritis may be aggravated by the anxiety, tension, and lack of distraction that follows bereavement.

However the previous relationship with the spouse was it is highly likely that it was the only close relationship left to the elderly person and so that need for that partner will be very great. Life outside the home tends to diminish as physical capabilities decline, and where there is chronic illness in one or both partners they will have relied on the other for practical care and support. The death of one may sometimes uncover great need and dependence of the remaining one, whose care had previously been provided totally by the dead partner.

Because the old do not have the long future alone to face up to, they have less incentive to relinquish their grief and may find a lot of comfort in trying to live as their partner would have wished. Statements such as 'I always did it like this because that's how he liked it' or 'I wouldn't want to join that group. My husband and I didn't like crowds' or 'He didn't like me going out in the evenings', which might cause some concern if made by a young person some time after bereavement, would be far less likely to be unhelpful for an elderly bereaved person. For them this may be a good way of coping and living with their loss. It may be particularly helpful for an elderly person to have a special place in the home or garden where they feel they can go and 'talk' to their partner. I have known many who have kept a special corner of the living room, for example, with a photograph and some flowers, or an area of garden with the deceased person's favourite plants or tree. Some of them have been relieved to know how this is not an unusual or unhealthy thing to do and that it can be comforting to 'talk' to the partner. Many elderly people are afraid to say they do this in case it is considered strange or a sign of mental illness.

Some elderly people have also expressed guilt because they have wanted to keep their partner's possessions intact and family members and others have suggested that this is morbid behaviour. It would appear that the need to retain precious reminders of their loved one and life together is, in fact, usual and healthy behaviour. There may sometimes be ulterior motives behind the suggestion that they should clear out and give away personal items belonging to their partner.

BEREAVED ELDERLY PARENTS

The elderly are, in particular, likely to benefit from volunteer support. Regular contact and availability is as important as responding to crises and any community schemes that help the elderly person to feel valued and relieve isolation are going to be helpful in the long term.

The following account of the loss of an elderly mother is a sensitive account of a common experience.

'Remembered with love'

I have worked with elderly people and studied the ageing process, revering the old for what they have been, rather than that they are has-beens, but how I resented it all happening to my 88-year-old mum. The restless plucking fingers, the wavering hand picking cobwebs from the air, the rheumy eyes, the lack of fastidiousness and self-preoccupation, which was so uncharacteristic and only applied to other people.

I looked after my mother for some months since her independent life was no longer possible, stimulating and encouraging the shreds of independence that remained.

Then one day she felt sick – 'Don't put her to bed', said the doctor 'or she will never get up', so for three days we struggled into clothes, girdle, stockings, the lot, until the exhaustion that followed seemed ridiculous. We succumbed to dressing gown and sitting out for a time but eventually bed took over and what relief she experienced. She felt sick and only wanted water and sleep and to be left alone.

'Feed her,' they said. 'Get her up,' they said. 'Walk her round the room,' they said. 'She'll use up the use of her legs.' 'If you are not doing all this you are not coping,' they said.

'She must drink,' they said. 'Look how dry her skin is.' But they did not tell you how to force fluids into an old lady who would lie comatose for hours at a time – also there was the ever-present thought that what goes in must come out!

I said, 'My mother is dying. Can't we just keep her comfortable and leave her in peace.' People say the end will come all in God's good time, oh no, it is often in man's good time; after modern theories have been put into practice life can be maintained long after any quality remains.

She gave us lots of frights when I summoned the family, then she rallied and lived to fight many more days. So often I wished, as I saw her sleeping peacefully, that she could just slip away – and then that terrible reaction, 'I have just wished my mother to be dead.'

I had wonderful support from doctor, community nurses, agency nurses from a private caring organization, the members of which became like family. They breezed in with their bright scarves, smiling faces from the outside world. The main difficulty was remembering all their names as a procession of Beryls, Helens and Annes crossed our threshold, all inspected by the family dog. I placed a photograph of my mother in a prominent place in the bedroom to remind me, and all the other carers, that she had not always been a demanding old lady.

Lifting her was the major problem and her bodily needs did not always coincide with the arrival of helpers so there were many hazardous exits between bed and commode, sometimes assisted by my husband, and I saw the last shred of my mother's dignity disappear.

One minor stroke followed another, each depleting her a little more. When her speech had gone she developed expressive eyebrows but we could not always understand what she tried to convey to us in anguish. I had not experienced death close at hand but the signs of the approaching end were unmistakable. I was there holding her hand, as I wanted, but did she know that I was there or was she already on the journey that one can only take alone? As her breaths got lighter she curled her lip and looked different – I wanted to say, like a child, 'Don't pull that face, mummy, it doesn't look like you'.

There were the arrangements to be made, the details of which suddenly became very important and the short service to be staged-managed. Although he did not know her well, the vicar spoke of mother as the gracious lady she was, my sister and I managed one voice between us during her favourite hymn, cracking on different verses. The flowers were lovely – she wanted flowers – and we returned home to yet more from friends who preferred to send them to the living. The comfort of this cannot be denied.

At a later date we took mother's ashes back to Birmingham for another service, which was attended by family who had not been able to travel south and the closest knit friends and neighbours who had been part of her life for so long. Her final resting place was with her parents in a corner of the churchyard and I felt a new peace that she was back where she belonged.

I was used to mother being away so that I did not feel a great miss from my daily life, but telling her things – that was and still is the big miss. I had written to her most weeks of my married life and all of a sudden all the little anedotes, family news, good and bad, hung in the air, untold. What would have pleased her still gives me pleasure.

The next stage was clearing mother's house, once it had been sold. We called in valuers who were either brash or denigrating when we longed for them to be respectful of the treasured pieces we had known for so long.

There were letters – from an old boyfriend who mother would have married but for his death in after the first world war, daily letters (sometimes sent and received the same day) containing what would now be said on the telephone. Those to and from our father confirming his lasting devotion were the most moving of all. We could not imagine him as 'laddie' or 'my boy' or our mother as 'giddy', full of fun and enjoying 'clicking' with the boys. There were poems written to each other and many expressions of love. I was a honeymoon baby and my arrival coincided with a financial disaster when they had to be parted. The letters of that time reflect the problems encountered and the hard times of their early marriage.

It was revealed, in familiar but much stronger handwriting, that milk for me cost 5/- a week, 12/6 was given to grandmother for board and lodging and a plea for another 2/6 as mother was hungry all the time! There were letters of congratulations at my birth and a calendar tear off for 27th April saying Red Letter Day!

Which leads me into clothes, still holding mother's shape, aura and most moving of all, the odd hanky in a pocket. The evening dresses and hats recalled many special occasions when elbow length gloves were essential – did her hand ever fit into those narrow gloves and fingers manipulate those tiny pearl buttons? The button box was another memory jerker, reminding us of linen shirt buttons and dresses from years back.

What happened to mother's possessions became very important to us, and as we stood in the empty rooms, we hoped she would be pleased where the things had 'gone' and that she will live on for family and friends. Immortality has many guises.

(reproduced with kind permission of Mrs Peggy Williams, 1989)

Outliving an adult child turns over the expected order of things and is likely to have as great an impact on the elderly as losing a child in younger years. This must be borne in mind when nursing elderly patients, for it is still easy to perceive them as old people and to forget that they may still be husbands and wives, mothers and fathers, brothers and sisters. Lesher and Berger (1988) studied 18 bereaved elderly mothers and found a high level of psychological distress.

LOSS THROUGH VIOLENCE

Death by violence adds another dimension to that universal and highly stressful experience of loss. An important element is the unexpectedness of it, which precludes any anticipatory grieving. The basic trust in other human beings with which most of us live our everyday lives is severely undermined.

Davidson (1984) describes the wars in which Israel has been involved and numbers 20,000 young men as having died in them, so he estimates there are about 20,000 bereaved families in Israel. For many years, he writes, there was an avoidance and denial within that culture, which he sees as being comparable to the reactions to the holocaust experiences during the first years of the Israeli state, an avoidance sustained by the strong desire to build for the future and to defend the new state and its security. The constant danger to security meant that a high public morale had to be maintained so behaviour tended to be stoical and deritualized, apart from widespread participation in national Remembrance Days. Attitudes and behaviour changes occurred after the 1973 war, and it was then that a network of formal and informal support began to supplement the previous concern with economic and practical needs.

Formal support was provided by notification teams, which informed families of their loss and then gave immediate support. One can easily imagine the stress of all those living on a special street, at the arrival of these teams. Their aims was to 'humanize a tragic event', by maintaining contact with the family, and visiting them regularly. They were, Davidson feels, highly significant, not least because, in common with war widows and bereaved parents in general, there is a strong need to be associated with the representative of the institution that gives meaning to the loss, for example the army, navy or air force, the Ministry of Defence, etc.

Within this general group of at risk bereaved people, Davidson points out that the high risk widows are those who do not ask for help or know how to ask for it, and yet seem to need it most, and those women who are most passive and have low self-esteem. Bereaved parents who are socially isolated, that is with no extended family, are also highly at risk. He also draws our attention to the bereaved father who receives less attention and is expected to be stoical. The death of his son in the war questions his value systems and identity and may throw into controversy the whole reason for living. For Jewish people there is an additional aspect to consider. When his father dies, his son recites the Kaddish prayer for him, as a symbol of life. If the son dies first, then this possibility of his own continuation has been lost, and creates an added dimension to the grief experienced.

Davidson's important point is that receiving recognition and consensus validates suffering, and what he refers to as a 'significant community' promotes positive coping responses, reduces negative reactions and so protects against the development of adverse later reactions. Although this is related to a country at war, there are some obvious implications for other kinds of bereavement within our own culture. The creation of a community that is significant to a particular group of bereaved people can sometimes be provided via self-help groups. The recognition of the uniqueness and value of each individual which we, as nurses, may strive to convey to patients and their families may go some way towards helping the bereaved to find meaning and ultimately, some kind of validation of their experience which can help later acceptance.

The Hungerford massacre in 1987 was death on a scale that we associate with the United States rather than England. This experience of community violence dramatically disrupts local life and is deeply disturbing to those living in the vicinity and also has an impact on others who read and hear about it in the news.

Kathi Nader (1987), looking at the impact of community violence from an American perspective, reports that individuals demonstrate a reduced energy for normal daily functioning, and disturbing changes in their thought patterns and behaviours. Reactions include psychological trauma, grief, worry about a significant other, and disruption of family and community function. She points out that everyone in the community is affected, not only the victim themselves and their families but also the rescue workers, policemen, ambulancemen and firemen.

Fear of the violence recurring can have a debilitating effect on individuals and the community at large. Children's responses are similar to adults', being influenced by age and developmental level. Both describe the repeated intrusion of disturbing thoughts, images and sounds and tend to dream about the violent event. Children experience a sense of isolation and lack of interest in their usual activities while adults describe their feelings as numb.

Immediately after the violent event, individuals describe increased states of arousal, including startle reactions, sleep disturbances and hypervigilance. They may feel a fear of specific locations, objects and human behaviours that remind them of the incident; they may also feel a more generalized sense of fear at moments of vulnerability, when alone in the bathroom, for example, or when going to bed.

How then, can the people of Hungerford and other communities exposed to violence be helped to cope? Nader outlines the ways of providing support via individual, family, classroom, group and community interventions. Individual treatment must explore the subjective experience of the violence. Intervention at the community level takes into account the need to integrate traumatized and bereaved people back into their jobs, classroom, etc. and this is a very critical step in the process of recovery. Group work is found to be an effective method of grief resolution.

Although symptoms may be better disguised and less obvious after the first year, she asserts that studies of both adults and children in the United States of America have shown that the persistence of post-traumatic stress symptoms years after the event continues without effective treatment.

DEATH FROM A DISASTER

When a sudden death happens as a result of some major disaster there are special problems, as was identified by work with the bereaved families of the 56 people who died in the fire at the Bradford City football match in 1986. Research cited by Wendy Harrison (1987), the Bradford fire coordinator, suggested that disaster victims are vulnerable to long-term emotional and psychological disturbances because disaster violates the predictable patterns of life, destroying the sense of safety and continuity that individuals need to make sense of life, accomplish everyday tasks and explore new kinds of experience with confidence. There are obvious parallels here with the feelings that accompany other kinds of unexpected death.

Harrison argues the need for supportive structures within the community if the crisis is to be resolved, and she quotes a research study by Erikson (1976) on the effects of a disaster on the people of Buffalo Creek in the USA. This consisted of a number of closely knit communities spread round a valley with a mountain tip overshadowing it. One day this tip overflowed, sweeping through the valley and 'consuming all that was in its path'. Those who survived were put into temporary accommodation, isolated from other friends and relatives. Two years later they were found to have made little recovery and it was suggested that this was due as much to the isolation from family and friends as to the horrific experience of the flood.

There appear to be implications here for the care of the groups of bereaved people, particularly those who are coming to terms with the sense of unreality that accompanies a sudden death. This leads to a marked need to ask many questions of those who were present at the death, yet sometimes health professionals and others are tempted to withhold some information in order to protect the bereaved person. It may well be that these half-truths contribute to the bereaved person's inability to make what happened seem real and permanent; they may dimly feel they are being fobbed off in some way.

BRAIN DEATH

Until the 1950s, conventional death was the only known kind. Since then the use of technology has enabled other bodily functions to be continued by machine – all, that is, except those performed by the brain. After brain stem testing, switching off a ventilator is an acceptance by staff that death has *already* taken place. Yet the family are faced with the body of the person they loved who may appear to them to be still very much alive. Therefore time is needed both to prepare the relatives and to support them for as long as they wish to stay.

Approaching the relatives about possible organ donation needs to be made when there is plenty of time for all options to be considered, so that they do not feel pressurized. Therefore, early contact with the local transplant coordinator is very helpful.

OTHER DEATHS IN INTENSIVE CARE

As in other acute settings, the environment emphasizes the drama of the situation and can make the loved person seem remote and dehumanized. The work is intense and dramatic, the temperature hot and sticky and the loved one is surrounded by complicated and alien equipment. 'She didn't look like my mother any more!' commented a friend whose mother had a severe myocardial infarction.

The demands of caring for many very ill patients may mean that the needs of the family have to take a lower priority. Therefore, the nurse has a hard task to bring warmth and caring into this atmosphere, to humanize it so that the relatives will remember the last moments in this way. Final goodbyes are particularly important and adequate time must be made available for this. A blessing from the chaplain, their own minister or a member of staff can, as in other wards, be of great comfort.

AIDS

Aids (acquired immune deficiency syndrome) is part of a spectrum of disease caused by HIV (human immunodeficiency virus) infection. It causes impairment of the body's immune system which can result in infection by organisms that usually have a low pathogenicity, so-called opportunistic infections.

The title of the *Sunday Times* colour supplement (21 June 1987), 'This issue is about Aids, and is also about You', hints at the difficulties experienced by those trying to promote prevention and understanding of this syndrome, namely the widespread beliefs that it affects only homosexuals and also that it is primarily an American problem. This fallacy affects the attitudes and, therefore, the behaviour of society to those who suffer from Aids and their families.

When the partner of the person dying of Aids is homosexual, his needs should be accepted by the nursing staff involved and the nature of the relationship must be acknowledged. They also need to be aware of the tremendous amount of fear that the gay partner will be experiencing. Their sexuality puts them at high risk, and having a lover who died of Aids serves to underline this. Therefore, they are likely to be preoccupied with their state of health and, when newly bereaved, can easily imagine that every physical symptom is an early sign of Aids. It may be useful to point out to them that many symptoms are commonly felt after the kinds of loss and stress.

However, it is also of obvious importance to encourage regular check-ups with their general practitioner or local clinic, and these may also help to relieve their anxieties. Gay men are accustomed to some extent in forming a minority group within society and many have strong networks of support within this group. The self-help support group can therefore be particularly appropriate.

The closeness and support of the gay community is well described by Adam Mars-Jones, who, suffering from Aids, is being cared for by two friends he had not even known before he had the disease. He writes:

> Diagnosis broke me up, the way a plough breaks earth, and all the recent growth, rooted so lightly, was pulled right up. But I was left ready for seeding when they phoned . . . . [these two comparative strangers]. I remember I said, 'Let's get one thing straight. I have never depended on the kindness of strangers.' Then I had to break it to them that what I was saying was 'Yes'.

The stigma of having Aids may create a growing number of people who grieve in secret or who hide the diagnosis from their family and friends, leading to complications during bereavement. For example, I know of a mother whose son died of Aids who was unable to share with anyone among her friends the true cause of his death. Working for a large organization most people knew her or of her and offered sympathy when she told them her only son was dying of cancer. A few months later, a close colleague in her department found that her son had cancer and inevitably wanted to discuss treatments and the course of the disease with this lady. She now faces the prospect of being 'found out' and the anguish and fear she feels is profound. She will need a lot of professional help to come to terms with the truth herself before she is able to be honest with those closest to her, and stop living a lie. This illustrates the problems of adjusting to bereavement where there is a high degree of anger against the one who died. There may be guilt over who they were and what they did, coupled with fear that this will be discovered by others.

This is a particular problem for wives whose husbands have died of Aids. The difficulties of caring for a bisexual patient dying of Aids who has both a wife and a long-term male partner are compounded by guilt and shame. The reality may come as a complete shock to the wife or else confirm her worst fears. She may well feel that this indicates that she is a failure both sexually and in making relationships.

In this situation nurses can help a great deal by their attitude of respect and with sensitivity and tact. The calm acceptance of the reality conveys the feeling that the wife is not completely alone, others have come through even this traumatic experience. Nurses also need to help the wife who may also be infected with HIV, and will need referral to the support and counselling services that are available for all HIV-infected people.

Much of the media coverage of Aids has used the word 'victim' when describing the sufferer, a word also often used when discussing cancer. The partner and/or family of the Aids patient are also victims because of the stigma attached to this kind of death. Yet, personally, I have a dislike of this word 'victim', which seems to suggest a powerlessness and hopelessness about that person or group. To me it conveys a subtle rejection of that person. Aids has created much fear among the general population and, as nurses, we have much to do to alleviate that fear and perpetuate a different attitude. It is, after all, one of the hallmarks of the caring profession such as ours that we accept people for who they are and what they are, without moral judgements.

Support to partners, families and friends both before and after the death of an individual with Aids can also be provided by Aids support groups that exist all over the country, a form of the Buddy system of help offered by the Terrence Higgins Trust. This was formed in 1982 by the friends of the first man to die in Britain of this syndrome. Buddies are volunteers, mostly gay men, who befriend the Aids patient and those he cares about both during the illness and afterwards. Newly diagnosed patients can be referred by the doctor or nursing staff to their local group, which cannot contact them until the referral has been made. After the death of an Aids patient, it is usual for the volunteer to take at least a month off. As with other kinds of support systems, a great advantage is that the volunteer can be seen to be unbiased, an outsider with no personal 'axe to grind'. The patient and family can use them as a sounding board, to discuss feelings and practical arrangements such as the funeral. Most Aids patients want to make specific instructions as to the type of funeral and burial that they want. This may, as in other situations, be different from what the family and friends want to happen. The volunteer and/or nursing staff may be involved in helping them to reach a compromise.

Knowledge can help to fight prejudice and reduce fear. Consider this example of unncessary fear that left a mother and son isolated from each other, even though he was dying. The family house was in an ordinary suburban street. Only round the corner in the next road, approximately 20 houses away was a house converted into several flats where this lady's son, aged 25, was dying of Aids, looked after effectively and caringly by his small circle of friends. They encouraged his mother to visit but she was unable to do so, because of the fear of catching it and of the neighbours finding out her son had Aids. The only way she could express her love for her son was by cooking him lunches while his friends were at work. These she carried to the door of his home in her shopping basket and then left on the step for him. It was certainly helpful to her later that she had at least done this for him, but she had felt extreme guilt and anxiety since his death.

When a son dies of Aids, whether he is gay, a drug addict or part of the heterosexual community, it would appear that fathers are less involved, they are often at work and tend to leave the caring both practically and emotionally to the women. (There are of course some notable exceptions to this generalization.) Where the son is gay, it may of course be more difficult for the father to accept reality and treat him as the individual he is.

It is evident that the principles of caring for Aids patients and their families has much in common with those of the palliative care movement, directed in the main towards cancer patients and their families. There appear to be parallels between Aids and cancer, such as marked fear of the disease, the mystery of it, the potential danger of quality as well as quantity of life, the sense of stigma and of being punished for past behaviours.

MENTAL HANDICAP

Grief following the death of a relative or friend is a very common and normal reaction for everyone, and that includes the mentally handicapped person. Although the help given by 'bereavement counselling' is now generally recognized, the grief of people who are mentally handicapped is not always acknowledged. They require support at this time of crisis in the same way as anyone else.

They may be in particular need for help if they have always spent their lives at home with their parents and had little or no preparation for the changes that the death of a parent will bring.

Neighbours, friends, relatives and professionals may themselves need help in supporting a mentally handicapped person at this time of grief and crisis. Those who are going to be very closely involved in trying to help may also need guidance to gain insight into the problems of the mentally handicapped. Staff may feel anxiety as they try to help and wonder how much the mentally handicapped person needs to know, what sort of explanations can be given and how far the mentally handicapped person's right to know should be respected. They may be distressed as they help the bereaved person and share with them the enormity of their loss. It is not easy to talk about death, and, if the mentally handicapped person is also very dependent and has special problems due to lack of speech, blindness, deafness or physical incapacity, the carer might feel even more at a loss to know how they can most sensitively be helped.

In this chapter we have looked at some of the groups of adults who may have particular problems during bereavement. It is necessary, however, to reiterate an earlier point, namely that it is possible to end up by allocating practically every bereaved person to an at risk group! However, when liaising between hospital and community and when planning any kind of help for bereaved people, a consideration of at risk groups is, I suggest, a necessary first step.

REFERENCES

Davidson, S. (1984) Families bereaved by war, holocaust and terrorism in Israel, *Bereavement Care*, Vol. 3(1).
Erikson, K. T. (1976) *In the Wake of the Flood*. Allen and Unwin, London.
Green, Michael (1985) *Loss of Old Age. In Loss: Proceedings of the BASW*

Summer School on Loss. British Association of Social Workers, June 1985.

Harrison, Wendy (1987) After the Bradford fire, *Bereavement Care.*

Lake, Tony (1984) *Living with Grief,* Sheldon Press, London.

Lesher, E. L. and Berger, K. J. (1988) Bereaved elderly mothers: changes in health, functional activities, family cohesion and psychological well-being. *International Journal of Aging and Human Development,* Vol. 26(2).

Mars-Jones, Adam (1988) Remission. *Granta Magazine,* Cambridge.

Moore, Ian (1986) Ending it all. *Nursing Times,* Vol. 82(7), pp. 48–9, 12 February.

Murray, Peter (1983) A suicide in the family. *The Times,* 1 June.

Nader, Kathi (1987) Hungerford's aftermath. *Nursing Times,* Vol. 83(36), pp. 20–2, 9 September.

Oakley, Ann (1985) *Taking it Like a Woman,* Penguin, London.

Oswin, Maureen (1981) *Bereavement and Mentally Handicapped People,* King's Fund Report (December).

Parkes, C.M. (1970) The first year of bereavement: a longitudinal study of the reaction of London widows to the death of their husbands, *Psychiatry,* Vol. 33, p. 44.

Parkes, C. M. and Weiss, R. S. (1983) *Recovery from Bereavement,* Basic Books Inc., New York.

Stengel, E. (1969) *Suicide and Attempted Suicide,* Pelican, London.

Torrie, Margaret (1975) *Begin Again: A Book for Women Alone,* Dent, London.

8. Family Needs after the Death

A man's dying is more the survivor's affair than his own.

Thomas Mann (1875–1955)

INTRODUCTION

In this chapter we consider the needs of bereaved people after the death, but how do we know what the needs of anyone may be? First of all, we look at expressed needs, checking the demands made on existing bereavement services. For example, the Christchurch Macmillan Unit offered a follow-up service to every close relative of every patient dying either in the Unit or at home. These visits were made by the home care nurses, the medical social worker and eventually by one or two volunteers. As time went on it became impossible to provide this for everyone and so we experimented with a personal letter that was sent to each relative not considered to be at risk and unlikely to receive any other outside support. Each letter was individually written and signed by the nurse sending it. Here is an example:

> Dr - - - has told me of your sad loss and we wondered how you were getting on now. My name is Jenny (Christian names were always used and professional titles omitted), and I would be happy to come and see you if you feel I could help in any way. Please don't hesitate to ring or write if I can do so. With best wishes from us all . . . .
> Yours sincerely, ...

The responses to these letters were very positive, with many recipients expressing enhanced feelings of security, 'It's so good to know I could talk to someone if I wanted to', 'I no longer feel so alone', 'It cheered me to know you had not forgotten me', 'I feel it would help me a lot if you could spare the time to answer my questions'. An average of 48 per cent requested contact with the writer either by telephone or, more commonly, via a home visit. Although the numbers at the time were too small to draw any valid conclusions, the reponse seemed to indicate that many bereaved people had needs that were not being met, and those who did receive follow-up were only the tip of an iceberg of unhappiness and isolation, whose needs were not being met by society in other ways.

Bereavement is a time of enormous, but usually unwanted, change.

IDENTIFYING BASIC NEEDS

Need for security

We have seen how bereavement undermines the basic faith and trust that most of us carry with us all our lives. We cannot provide security for anyone else, although some people try to do this by overprotecting the vulnerable or by making themselves indispensable, which is meeting their own needs and not those of the bereaved person. The only way any of us can feel really secure is to realize that the most effective support is ourselves. Relying on others always means that, for one reason or another, they could let us down. The way we think undoubtedly determines how we feel and so the rasing of our self-esteem, the expectation from others that we will be able to cope plus practical strategies for dealing with problems will all help the bereaved person to feel they can support themselves.

Need for physical health and fitness

This is so often overlooked even by nurses, yet we know that standards of physical fitness are related to the individual's ability to cope with stress of many kinds. Information about such aspects as healthy eating, exercise plans and relaxation techniques, provided that this is geared to a consideration of the individual's lifestyle, can be very welcome and also, indirectly, meet the need for security by communicating the message that the bereaved individual is a valued person who should be taking care of themselves. Discussion about these needs can be followed by recommending books and tapes from the local library and where groups or classes meet that the bereaved person might be interested in attending later on. For example, I know of a number of widows who have benefited greatly from joining a very good local yoga class.

Need to cope with vulnerable times

It can be helpful in preventing problems, to discuss with the bereaved person their own personal low points and help them, wherever possible, to work out a strategy to help them through them. Difficult days that seem to be shared by most bereaved people are Sundays, Bank Holidays and anniversary of all kinds, from Christmas and birthdays to the anniversary of when the loved one died. There may be others associated with activities done together, shared treats, times of the year when holidays were taken or visits made to others. It is often possible, when exploring their lifestyle, to help them see how it could be rearranged or activities extended, so that they are not alone at those times. A practical way of overcoming the dread of a Sunday alone, and of missing the ritual of the Sunday roast dinner, was suggested by one lady who invited two or three other elderly people who were also alone for Sunday lunch. They arranged a rota between them, eating at each other's houses each week. The one widower in the group who never cooked before enjoyed this challenge enormously, spending the weekend before his 'turn' poring over recipe books and doing his shopping. It is important that these strategies are seen to come, as far as possible, from the bereaved people themselves rather than being outside suggestions, and that the visitor does not impose his own solutions that seem right to him but may be quite inappropriate for others.

Need for stability

We have already looked at the many facets of bereavement that contribute to feelings of instability and even loss of identity. There is, therefore, a great need for a stable base to counter these influences, and the individual's personal anchor points such as their home, job, routine and hobbies should, as far as possible, remain unchanged for the first few months as least. Yet there is a tendency for bereaved people to think that the major change that has been forced upon them should be accompanied by other drastic changes in their life. The possibility of moving house is often discussed, particularly if this is linked to the suggestion from family or friends that the bereaved person should move nearer to them or even in with them. Sometimes this is connected to a financial need to live more cheaply or to move to a smaller home with less maintenance and upkeep. There may be sound reasons for such a decision but it is still wise to encourage the bereaved person to wait a while. They are unlikely to be in the clear-headed state needed to evaluate proposed changes with such far-reaching consequences and these include retiring from a job, giving up a part-time or voluntary work routine, taking on a large commitment such as altering their house, or even staying away from their home for long periods. The latter strategy was adopted by a widow I knew who told me afterwards that it had been 'a big mistake. I was escaping from the reality I had to face. And I spoilt those weekends with my friend dreading all the time the thought of going back. When I finally faced going back to my house I was devastated but I came to realize that I could not start to live again until I had faced all those memories. I had tried to escape but you can't.'

Need for others

Most of us are sociable beings and have a need, at every level, for human contact and to be needed by others. The majority of people do want to help others and there are certainly rewards for those who help as well as for those who receive it. As nurses we know this, and we are often made to realize by our patients, as well as by their relatives, that it is often easier to be the giver rather than to be the recipient of care. It can, therefore, help bereaved people to explore what they feel they have to offer others in the community around them so that they have the dignity and self-esteem of being a helper and carer themselves. At the beginning of bereavement, they may need to be encouraged to accept help that is offered to them and even, in some circumstances, to be brave enough to ask for help. There is often an inclination to decline help and support offered, and this can be unfortunate because later when they may feel they would welcome those offers of support they may well no longer be forthcoming. So they may benefit from being encouraged to accept help and contact even though they may not feel like it at the time it is offered, and to consider what they feel they can give back later when they feel stronger.

Need for self-indulgence

This basic human need is one which, I feel, is often overlooked by many of us. We tend to expect rewards of any kind to be given to us by others, and to feel guilty if we treat ourselves in any way. This may not necessarily be about material things such as buying a lovely dress even though we do not really need it, or a book that catches our eye, or cream cakes to gorge on at teatime. It can also refer to giving ourselves time to visit an exhibition on the way home even though this makes the meal late for others, to staying up to watch the late-night film just because we want to. Few of us have been socialized into the idea that, on occasion, it is right for us to pamper ourselves or to reward ourselves for something we have done. Therefore to get this idea across to a bereaved person may be difficult and certainly requires an appropriate moment.

Nevertheless it can be very helpful, particularly for those who are alone, to feel comfortable about giving themselves the occasional reward or the regular pleasure of something they enjoy. What it actually is does not matter, as long as it makes the individual feel good – but not guilty! The widow of a solicitor I knew particularly dreaded visits to her late husband's offices. His colleagues could have visited her at home but she felt it was a challenge and wanted to prove to herself that she could cope. However, each time she went, she followed it with a reward of some kind such as inviting a friend to have lunch with her. These are very useful as reinforcement following a visit but can also go some way towards helping those who do not receive any other kind of support.

If we take a humanistic view, based on concern for the individual, we might view bereavement as being about the pursuit of personal growth and fulfilment, a process whereby each individual is responsible for himself as well as, in part, to others.

Maslow (1968) studied what motivated people in certain situations and noted that the results tended to fall into a certain pattern. These needs were inborn and the lower the need the stronger it was, lower needs having to be at least partially satisfied before the individual moved upwards to the next. He categorized them and arranged them in a hierarchial structure. His hierarchy of needs seems to have something to say to us when applied to the context of bereavement.

PHYSIOLOGICAL NEEDS

The most fundamental needs are for survival and for comfort. Therefore a bereaved person is threatened at this level because they often feel unable or unwilling to survive without the one who has died and they have also been reminded of the inevitability of their own death. Other physiological needs such as being able to sleep and eat are also affected by the emotional turmoil of bereavement.

OTHER NEEDS

Safety needs

In order to feel safe, an individual needs to be free of fear, yet bereavement is about facing many fears and anxieties. In one sense, perhaps none of us can ever find true safety for as long as we are reliant on others we can always be let down, and if we rely only on ourselves we can still let ourselves down! Taking responsibility for oneself can enhance feelings of security.

Love and belonging need

In this context these are about the need to be understood and valued as a separate being and to be accepted as such by others, as well as by one or two special people. This is to do with feelings of community where each person can participate and give to others as well as receiving support from them. Individual contributions are valued. When searching for meaning and a new way of living, bereaved people may feel they have nothing to offer to others and that they are not understood or valued. If they feel unable to give anything of themselves to anyone or a group of people, this lowers self-worth and dignity. 'Might as well be thrown on the scrap-heap,' said one widow. 'People are very kind to me but they don't want anything from me.'

Self-esteem and esteem by others

As well as a stage this can be seen as a thread running through this classification. Feelings of competence and accomplishment are important to all of us and our roles in society need to be recognized and so endorsed by others. Bereaved people, especially when elderly, may sometimes feel they are treated as objects of pity and little respect is accorded them for their previous roles and status.

Cognitive needs

This refers to the need for knowledge, for making sense of the world and events that happen within it. The search for meaning has been mentioned previously and in a sense bereaved people are on a journey of making sense of their experiences, although they may be at different stages and some may even be refusing to begin.

Aesthetic needs

In everyone there is a capacity to appreciate the good and the beautiful although ideas as to what represents these notions may vary. For Jane, the young girl dying of cancer in Zorzka's *A Way to Die*, a single rose pinned to her nightdress and a piece of velvet to touch were what fulfilled her aesthetic needs. People undergoing the stress of bereavement often experience a heightened perception of both pleasant and unpleasant stimuli. Their tolerance levels for sensations such as loud noises, the incessant chatter of children, the sound of different music or the smell of food cooking may be unusually low. Sensations they find pleasant may, however, evoke deeper feelings than before and may also have an added poignancy if connected with memories of the person they have lost.

SELF-ACTUALIZATION

This is seen as the highest but weakest need. It refers to the individual's motivation to achieve their fullest potential and to find personal meaning in their life.

Behaviours that Maslow (1968) identified as leading to this stage included an ability to concentrate fully, a flexibility of outlook, a lack of pretension and the courage to give up defences. These, you may feel, are present in very young children and you may also have noticed them in some dying people, death being seen as birth in reverse. People become alone, dependent and innocent, having given up their usual defences.

It is possible to view bereavement as a path to self-knowledge. Many people do assert that there is no loss that cannot lead to gain. However, many bereaved people would still, if they had such a choice, do without personal growth! As Rabbi Harold Kushner (1981) wrote about the loss of his son after a long chronic illness,

> I am a more sensitive person, a more effective pastor, a more sympathetic counsellor because of Aaron's life and death than I would ever have been without it. And I would give up all these gains in a second if I could have my son back. If I could choose, I would forego all the spiritual growth and depth which has come my way because of our experiences, and be what I was fifteen years ago, an average Rabbi, an indifferent counsellor, helping some people and unable to help others, and the father of a bright, happy boy. But I cannot choose.

Having looked at the possible needs of the family after the death, we will now turn to the many ways in which we may be able to help, either directly or by initiating support and information.

REFERENCES

Kushner, Rabbi Harold (1981) *When Bad Things Happen to Good People*, Shocken Books, New York.

Maslow, Abraham H. (1968) *Motivation and Personality*, Harper and Row, New York.

Zorzka, R. and V. (1980) *A Way to Die: Living to the End*, Deutsch, London.

9. What Can We Do To Help?: Care in the Community

Give sorrow words: The grief that does not speak knits up the o'erwrought heart and bids it break.

William Shakespeare (1564-1616)

INTRODUCTION

Each of us belongs to many communities. The area in which we belong, the social groups with which we share our leisure, and those with a similar spiritual philosophy are all examples of communities.

When working outside hospital, nurses make up their own community profile in order to understand and describe the area in which they work.

Hubley (1982) suggests that the following information needs to be gathered to make up such a profile (Table 9.1). This appears to be helpful when considering the needs of bereaved people, by understanding the context in which they live.

There are, of course, some significant differences in caring for people at home rather than in hospital, and these apply to the care of relatives as well as patients. Those taking on a helping role (whether nurses or others) need to be aware that:

- Whoever visits does so as a guest.
- They have no right of entry.

Table 9.1 Community information

Environment	Geography, urban/rural, transport, land use, recreational facilities, housing
History	History of area, activities of local groups, issues of special interest from newspapers
Residents Basic	Total population, age distribution, children under fourteen years; population 65 years, preschool, turnover of population, birth rate, family sizes, vulnerable groups, such as single-parent families and handicapped, ethnicity, religion, social class, employment
Health and social welfare	Utilization of hospitals/clinics/general practitioners, social services uptake, free school meals, data on community health from local health service records or other sources (exact nature of data will depend on special interests of health educator making community profile)
Perceptions of area	Residents' perceptions of problems of area; attitudes towards other residents, agencies, officials, local politicians; attitudes and beliefs concerning health and felt needs for health education and health care services

- They need to be fully aware of the vast range of resources that exist in their own particular area, some of which may be unique to it.
- However good their intentions, they *may* not be acceptable to the bereaved person who is free to reject their offers of support.
- Their aim must be to assist the bereaved person to cope both emotionally or practically in their absence.
- When the helper has built a relationship over a period of time, friendships can develop; the complications of this possibility need to be thought through at the beginning.

The quality of the links between the hospital and the community are always of crucial importance to patient and family care. When the family of the dying patient can see the two working closely together they can feel comfort and security from the caring professions.

These links have to be worked at by both hospital and community-based staff. Knowledge and understanding of each other's roles encourages mutual respect. Well-developed communication skills enable assessment of the family's needs to be passed on to those caring for them at home.

Most of us, when working in hospital, have watched relatives leaving the ward after the patient's death, and felt concerned as to how they would manage. It is usually the nurse in charge who assesses their probable needs and supplies the community staff with information that will be helpful to them. With unexpected death it is obviously vital that this *information be passed on quickly*. There are few of us who have worked in the community who have not, at some time, appeared on a bereaved person's doorstep without knowing that a death has taken place.

SERVICES INVOLVED IN BEREAVEMENT SUPPORT

Nurses are just one group of professional people who may be involved in bereavement via specialists such as the Macmillan and hospice home care teams, community nursing sisters and district enrolled nurses, health visitors and liaison sisters. The notion of helping people in need is a prime motivation for people who work in all aspects of health care. In the past this help has tended to be provided for bereaved people by their own families and by other members of small communities, because in such communities people are interdependent. This support has been supplemented at various times by members of religious orders, and more recently, via various statutory services. In our society help for a host of people in need including the ill, the handicapped, the poor, the elderly, as well as bereaved people, tended to become the province of professionals or 'experts'.

Table 9.2 shows what may appear to be a bewildering range of services in the community involved in bereavement support.

THE PRIMARY HEALTH CARE TEAM

Within the multidisciplinary primary health care team is the nursing team made up of district nurses, district enrolled nurses and auxiliaries, health visitors and practice nurses.

The district nursing sister

Her chief responsibility is to decide on the nursing care each patient needs and to ensure that it is carried out. She is leader of the team that includes district enrolled nurses and nursing auxiliaries. The nature of her work

Table 9.2 Community services

The primary health care team
General practitioner
District nursing officer
Health visitor
Practice nurse
Midwife
Specialist community nurse
Community psychiatric nurse
Administrative support

Social services
Social worker – generic or specialist (sometimes attached to the primary health
   care team)
Home help
Meals-on-wheels
The provision of aids and adaptations

Department of Social Security
Financial advice and provision of benefits

Voluntary organizations
Self-help groups
Neighbourhood schemes, such as 'street wardens'
Church groups
Volunteers attached to primary health care teams (for example, caring for the
   elderly)

---

often brings her into close relationships with patients and families. She
will care for the dying patient at home and be able to provide continuity
of care by supporting the family afterwards.

The health visitor

She is a registered nurse who has undergone further training for the
Certificate in Health Visiting. Although her main focus is on the health
and development of babies and children up to school age, she is considered to be a family visitor. As such she is increasingly involved in meeting
the needs of elderly people. Therefore she is likely to be involved in
supporting both bereaved parents and older bereaved people.

Practice nurses

These nurses are employed primarily to work in treatment rooms in general practices, using practical nursing procedures, screening tests and giving health advice. Their work may sometimes give them the opportunity to offer practical and emotional support to bereaved people visiting the practice.

The wider nursing team is made up of midwives, specialist nurses, hospital nurses and volunteers.

Midwives

They provide both antenatal and postnatal care in conjunction with the general practitioner and hospital maternity services. They are, of course, closely involved in the care of the newborn baby. In this role they have a valuable part in supporting the family whose baby dies around the time of birth.

Specialist nurses

These include many nurses working in the community or in liaison roles between hospital and community. They have expertise in a particular area, and can be used as a resource by others as their knowledge is up to date and backed up by experience. These include Macmillan and hospice-based home care nurses, community psychiatric nurses and community mental handicap nurses. All these should have expertise in supporting bereaved children and adults.

School nurses, specialist paediatric nurses and stoma nurses are examples of other community-based nurses who may, at times, need to help in supporting bereaved families.

Liaison nurses

These are hospital-based but are appointed to promote continuity of care between hospitals and community. In this role they may sometimes be involved with distressed relatives of a patient who has died in hospital.

Any or several of these people or groups may be involved in providing bereavement support. Perhaps surprisingly, having viewed these extensive lists, you may find that some bereaved who do need help do not receive it at all! A few may have too much help offered and then, as in similar situations in the community, it is necessary for nurses (and others) to recognize this and know when to withdraw their help.

BEREAVEMENT SERVICES

The provision of services, whether professional or volunteer, are a response made to the needs of bereaved people on humanitarian grounds, but also for expediency. We know that the loss of an important emotional relationship is an event with a high risk of subsequent illness. For example, in a well-known study by Parkes (1970) there was found to be a 40 per cent higher death rate amongst the bereaved within six months of the loss than for a control group. The main cause of death was coronary artery disease, which in the past would have been referred to as 'dying of a broken heart', and this was most evident in widows.

Work by Parkes (1980), Vachon *et al.* (1980), Parkes and Parkes (1984) and others indicate that support to families prior to the death of the patient and afterwards is likely to have a beneficial effect on adjustment in the long term.

However, it can be argued that it is the responsibility of each individual to cope effectively with his predicament, drawing on previous experiences of loss and ways of coping which have proved to be effective for him. Should there be any need for outside interventions of any kind? I agree that for many people it is unnecessary, and in previous chapters we looked at some of the indicators and the groups that might be particularly at risk. Experience does tell us that there often is a need for help from outside the immediate family/friendship circle, and for some people of course this circle does not in fact exist.

PLANNING

Various issues must be considered when planning a support service for bereaved people:

(1) Time management: Can you still be efficient whilst aiming for flexibility of time that may be needed by any individual? When, and how often, do you intend to visit? Is there a maximum or minimum number of visits that can be made?

(2) Evaluation: How can you show your managers that such a preventive service is being effective?

(3) Quality control: Can you measure the support you give in any way?

(4) Accessibility: How will you decide who is to have access to this extra support? What are your criteria for those at risk?

(5) Liaison: Who else might you want to work with, as needed? (For example, minister, volunteer, self-help group etc.) It can be helpful to make contact *before* you start.

(6) Training: Would you need any extra training to help you in this role? (For example, interpersonal skills).

(7) Attitudes: Paternalistic/maternalistic attitudes are common: whose needs would you be meeting? Bereavement support can be very satisfying and there can be rewards for the helper who enjoys feeling needed. I remember occasions when I continued to support for too long, becoming a 'prop' to the bereaved person and finding it increasingly difficult to withdraw.

Potential problems

Potential problems when planning a bereavement service are:

(1) Time management: Bereavement visits can take a long time and it is obviously not possible to leave a person who has become distressed; it is often just when the nurse has her hand

	on the door knob or garden gate, when the bereaved person starts to tell them how they are really feeling.
(2) Priorities:	Bereavement visits tend to be low priority in comparison with other demands.
(3) Accessibility:	Contacting a bereaved person who is, for example, working and only available in the evenings or at weekends when staff are already in short supply.
(4) Cost and quality control:	Bereavement visiting by professionals is expensive and the quality may be variable.

These four points indicate the need for evaluation of both short-term and long-term outcomes of bereavement visiting.

Increasingly, bereavement services are becoming more formalized as caring people have become more aware of the needs and have looked at different ways of providing help to meet them. It is important for us know what kind of services do exist in our area. I am sure you could give examples of relatives of patients in hospital or in the community who have caused you concern and whom you have wanted to ensure would be followed up later on.

However, if we talk about 'follow-up', what do we really mean? Are we merely 'hedging our bets', making sure our professional responsibilities can be seen to have been handed on to others? What do we anticipate a follow-up service should do, and what role do we expect the individual to take, when doing it?

AIMS OF HELP IN BEREAVEMENT

Bereavement is one crisis situation where there is an enforced change. The usual options in such situations are:

(1) To try to change the situation.
(2) To adapt to the situation, in other words, to change oneself.
(3) To exit from the situation.
(4) To develop ways of living with the changed situation.

It is important for the helper to clarify with the bereaved person what they see as the purpose of any supportive visit. It would appear that in bereavement the individual is trying to:

(1) Understand themselves and their situation.
(2) Achieve change(s) in the way they are feeling and to feel confident again.
(3) Have the ability to make necessary decisions.
(4) Have the ability to confirm such decisions.
(5) Adjust to the situation because it is not going to change.
(6) Express and let go of feelings (alone or with others); feel able to cry and to stop crying.
(7) Examine all available options.
(8) Be able to share memories of the deceased person and their life together.

EVALUATION

Evaluation is the necessary last step of the helping process and it involves looking at both the outcome and the process involved at reaching it. The kinds of questions the helper has to ask include the following:

The outcome

(1) What were my aims and objectives?
(2) Did I achieve them?
(3) In the light of what happened, were my aims realistic?
(4) What were the bereaved person's expectations and objectives?
(5) Did they gain what they wanted? Were their expectations fulfilled?

The process

(6) Can I define the quality of the interview as a whole?
(7) What kinds of feelings were being expressed?
(8) How did I respond to them?
(9) Were there any silences? If so, what caused them?
(10) How comfortable was I with them?
(11) Did I fail to respond appropriately to any verbal or non-verbal cues?
(12) Did the interview draw to a close in a suitable way?
(13) Should I visit this person again?
(14) Should I involve any other person or service to support this person (with their permission)?

(15) Are there any changes I would make if doing this interview again?
(16) Do I need to talk this interview through with someone more experienced?
(17) Have I learnt something new about myself?

HELPING STRATEGIES

Observation skills are needed when visiting a bereaved person at home, and are fundamental to good nursing practice in any situation. It is useful for the bereavement visitor to have some kind of checklist to look at before and after the visit to assist in focusing on key areas (see p. 143). It will also be helpful when writing up the visit afterwards. It should never, of course, be taken into the home because evidence of paperwork interferes with the establishment of a relationship, and is likely to convey messages quite contrary to the kind of communication intended!

Various forms and checklists have been devised and it is probably best to adapt these, as experience dictates, to the individual style of the visitor. Checklists form one of several very useful ways of helping people to overcome problems, clarify options and achieve their own goals. To put it into perspective, Hopson (1982) distinguishes between six types of helping strategy, all of which we can as nurses use to good effect at appropriate times.

Giving advice

As nurses, we are frequently asked for advice and we try to give an informed opinion of the best course of action based on *our* view of the patient or family situation. When this is concerned with practicalities, such as financial problems, it is probably appropriate.

Giving information

We are constantly asked by relatives for information usually concerning the patient's current condition and likely prognosis or discharge date. Sometimes we are asked for other types of information such as who to go to for particular advice or the whereabouts of special agencies. We may be asked about legal or financial matters and we need to know to whom and how to refer the individual if we do not know the answer to their questions ourselves. We have discussed how a lack of information of any kind makes people feel vulnerable.

Direct action

Sometimes it is necessary to do something on behalf of someone else or to act immediately to provide for another's need. Intervening in a crisis is one of those occasions, and bereavement follow-up support may sometimes come under this category. A crisis is said to occur when something unexpected happens which calls into question an individual's base for reality and alternative meaning cannot readily be found. This puts the individual into an apparently alien chaotic world where this sense of self is lost. The hazardous event of bereavement constitutes a threat and there is no coping mechanism already in existence for the individual to enable him to quickly re-establish his equilibrium. Rapoport (1970) sees a crisis as an upset in a steady state with the associated stress of straining towards achieving a new equilibrium.

As nurses, we do sometimes have to take direct action to ensure that a distressed relative does not go home alone, to alert their general practitioner and the primary health care team to visit quickly if we feel they are at risk, to arrange for the social services to provide a meal or to give immediate help to a relative who appears to be unable to care for themselves.

Teaching

Teaching is increasingly becoming a major nursing responsibility. Although it, too, is about giving information it is much more than this. It is about passing on knowledge and skills to improve the quality of life of any individual and, for the bereaved relative, it may be about caring for themselves in order to improve their general health and raise self-esteem.

System change

This helping strategy is about working towards influencing and improving systems that are causing difficulties and conflicts to groups of people. In other words, it is about trying to change organizations and bureaucracies such as the National Health Service, rather than concentrating on trying to change individuals. This is not always viewed as a nursing responsibility. Indeed, we all tend to grumble about perceived shortcomings and injustices, but are not always motivated or skilled in knowing how to generate change by working together as a group. This does appear to be changing. It is an aspect of professionalism that individual nurses have to think through carefully before either accepting or rejecting this responsibility in any given situation.

Counselling

This will be discussed fully in Chapter 10. Counselling services may exist especially for bereaved people, but it is worth remembering that other listening/visiting services may also be useful, such as the Samaritans, Relate (formerly marriage guidance), well women centres and church groups.

SELF-HELP GROUPS

In recent years there has been a movement away from more orthodox and statutory services and towards various alternatives. This increased desire to take responsibility for oneself has in part caused a great increase in the number of self-help groups. There is a realization that the helping professions can never provide the amount of involvement and support that so many people desperately need. As Robinson (1979) pointed out, the natural support systems of our society such as the church, the neighbourhood and the family, are all in decline. The result is a search for feelings of community, by people who feel helpless or hopeless and without control over their lives. Self-help groups are not, however, mere refuges. They provide a very positive response to needs, providing mutual support for those who share a common problem, practical solutions to specific difficulties, and an opportunity for members to build a new set of relationships and even, for some, a new way of life.

Therefore, most groups aim to provide friendship and opportunities for socializing, practical advice and assistance when needed and, sometimes, a form of pressure group to lobby for political or legal changes which may be of benefit to members of the particular group.

The shared experience of coping with disease, disability and loss can help to minimize feelings of isolation. The fact that others are in the same position diminishes stress, and being able to meet others who have been through a similar experience and have adjusted to it helps to give confidence and a feeling of regaining control.

Information of a practical nature is also very helpful as is guidance on the array of welfare services and benefits to which the bereaved person may be entitled.

There are, however, problems in joining these groups. The onus is on the bereaved person to make the initial contact, and this can be very demanding. One lady said she was 'ridiculously nervous' about phoning such an organization even after being given the telephone numbers of two local members to contact. She put off telephoning for several days. It is daunting to ring a stranger and the effort requires a lot of emotional energy. It is also hard to join a group of strangers and may involve travelling to unfamiliar places, perhaps alone for the first time.

Also, many people are fundamentally 'non-joiners' while others feel that meeting other bereaved people would be 'morbid'. They may fear that it will be necessary to talk about their own experiences before they feel ready to do so.

Many bereaved people would agree with Schiff (1977) who, whilst recognizing that professional intervention might sometimes be helpful, still argues that the bereaved can best gain comfort, understanding and hope from others who have also been through the despair and recovery that follows loss. She writes of her own and her husband's attempts at helping other bereaved parents that, 'What we had was something few could give them. We had experience. When they saw us, they saw a mother and father of a dead child, who were able to cope.'

Cruse

One example of a self-help group is Cruse, the national association for widows, and now widowers as well. They put newly bereaved people in touch with others for mutual support and practical help. They run group meetings to provide friendship. They have a well-developed training programme for volunteers and run national conferences to create and maintain awareness of the needs of bereaved people. They also publish useful material, in particular their quarterly journal *Bereavement Care*, which contains articles and book reviews and other helpful updated information. Many widows and widowers I have met through Cruse groups tell me of the relief they feel at being comfortable about sharing their feelings with others who have been through a similar experience. 'I can't tell them they don't understand because they do!' said one widow.

Informal groups

Some groups have been started because those who attend have in common the loss of a loved one in a particular location. An example is the Pilgrim Club at St Christopher's Hospice in Sydenham, London, or the 'family evenings' run by many Macmillan units, which are informal opportunities for recently bereaved people to 'pop in' and talk to others. Although these less structured groups often provide an opportunity for relatives to talk about their experiences and feelings, they are also used as a way of sharing and obtaining information on many practical concerns. One satisfied gentleman told me at the end of one 'family evening' that he felt much better now he had been able to find out the criteria for being provided with a home help, the cheapest local plumber and the best way of making his favourite snack, an omelette!

Addresses of self-help organizations can be found in Appendix 1.

For nurses, it may be useful to think in terms of trying to reach bereaved people who are unsupported, by starting some kind of self-help group through existing services such as the primary health care team. For example, a health visitor, community nurse or community psychiatric nurse might consider starting one in their local area by obtaining the names of recently bereaved people from the general practitioner. The next step would be to look for indicators of at risk status, for example, age, existence of other family members, living alone, circumstances of the loss, etc. Then it would be necessary to find a meeting place, as accessible as possible, and to enlist some help to provide refreshments and help to create an informal and welcoming atmosphere. The nurse's role could probably be summed up as a facilitator, establishing contact between those needing help and those with time and resources to provide it. I would see the long-term aim as being to withdraw, having left group members with the skills and motivation to continue running the group and letting it evolve to meet the needs of newly bereaved people.

As we have already realized, these groups can only cater for the needs of a small number of bereaved people. Some will always refuse to be part of any group, some feel quite unable to meet a number of strangers no matter how friendly, some will tell us that they do not wish to meet others in the same position as themselves as they perceive this to be 'morbid' or 'depressing'. Many elderly or nervous individuals are unable to travel to a group and need help and companionship for such a journey, no matter how short and even during daylight. Most self-help groups will invariably provide this assistance, at the least during the first few meetings.

PRACTICAL HELP

All the support and sharing in the world cannot make up for the practical help that is needed by most bereaved people, at least at first. Financial advice and assistance may be needed, meals need to be cooked, lawns mowed and houses cleaned. These are always ways of showing support and warmth for people who find verbal communication difficult. An invitation to lunch, a pudding left on the doorstep, the lawn mowed (without asking) are all tangible expressions of caring.

Media

Booklets are also useful if available in public places where those in need can easily and unobtrusively pick them up. The local health centre, doctors' and dentists' waiting rooms, citizens advice bureaux, post offices and social security offices, adult education centres, churches and luncheon clubs are all examples of places where these items can be available. If they are not, it may be possible for the nurse to instigate this.

Local departments of health and social security and libraries keep stocks of DHSS leaflets on all the various benefits and pensions and they are able and willing to answer personal queries.

Libraries

Here it is possible to obtain books, tapes and videos that may be helpful. These also provide full information on the resources and activities available in the community. Many also operate a domiciliary service for housebound people. Bereaved people may not ask directly for this kind of help but, in my experience, many have shown interest when it has been suggested to them. Something that can be read, or watched or listened to in privacy at the moment it is wanted can be very useful. The bereaved person is then in control and can use them as they need.

Diaries

For some people, the use of a diary or notebook in which to record feelings and memories can be very therapeutic. It is a private outlet for negative thoughts and a way of charting progress. 'I realize now how much better I am feeling!' was one comment made with surprise by a lady who had been keeping a diary intermittently for six months. Sometimes a tape recorder is preferred.

Some people may be encouraged by recording their thoughts in order to share with, and help, others at a future date. It is another way of giving back, of feeling that your unique experience may be able to contribute some hope and comfort to someone else and/or help professionals or volunteers to be more effective in the support and services they can offer.

VOLUNTEER INVOLVEMENT

Many kinds of volunteers schemes exist in various parts of the country. Some of these are concerned with particular groups, such as the relatives of cancer patients, for example, volunteers attached to Sir Michael Sobell House, Oxford, who have a paid volunteer organizer and a well-structured system of volunteer training and support. Some are involved with particular client groups such as the elderly – for example, volunteers attached to general practices in the Bournemouth areas who visit elderly people often find they have problems which are associated with bereavement. Well-known groups of volunteers such as the Samaritans are also involved from time to time with people whose preoccupation with suicide has been brought about or exacerbated by a bereavement.

For those contemplating setting up some kind of service, the possibility of involving volunteers is an attractive one. However, there are some important factors to be considered. The selection of volunteers (and professionals for that matter) is obviously crucial. Criteria have to be formulated so that people appropriate to the task are chosen. An area of debate is whether people who are themselves bereaved should be accepted on to a programme or not. At first sight this may appear to be wholly desirable as those who have come through a similar experience should be able to establish a rapport and be able to respond more sensitively. This is, after all, a guiding principle behind self-help groups. Any difficulty lies in the length of time they have been bereaved and whether they have, in fact, resolved their grief or whether they are still working through it. If they are still undergoing a process of adjustment they may be unable to be objective enough to give hope to others. But when they have adjusted to their changed situation this is an invaluable strength when relating to and empathizing with others who are more recently bereaved. A strategy also needs to be worked out to help volunteers who are found at interview, or when actually involved in supporting bereaved people, to be unsuitable for whatever reason. It is important from the perspective of meeting the needs of the volunteers themselves that they should be helped to find fulfilling alternatives and that they should not be left with any feeling of personal failure or guilt.

A training programme of some kind needs to be planned to give volunteers guidelines and confidence and to enable them to meet each other and those who can be available to back up if necessary. Careful thought needs to be given as to where and when this should take place so that those without transport and those who dislike being out at night will still be able to attend. The content needs to include guidelines of what to look for, indicators of people who may be at risk and some participatory sessions to give practice in responding to difficult emotions such as anger, guilt or depression. It is essential to know clearly who to go to with queries or concerns and to have regular opportunities for discussion with others. Wherever possible, it is helpful for the volunteer to be able to observe visits with others who are more experienced and to be able to analyse these afterwards.

However, such services that have existed to help bereaved people have been very fragmented, so many if not most of those who might benefit do not receive any outside support. Professionally run and staffed services are expensive and there is bound to be conflict and controversy over priorities when allocating funds. For example, disagreement may well arise between specialist nurses or community nurses and their respective managers, as to the feasibility of providing bereavement services when caseloads are already large and overstretched. Bereavement visits may appear to be difficult to evaluate in terms of prevention of ill-health, longer-term primary health care team involvement or other measures of effectiveness. If they appear to be unstructured without clearcut objectives that can be measured there will be little opportunity to analyse the possible effectiveness of the work. Furthermore, to be worthwhile, visits may need to be lengthy and certainly they are likely to be demanding of the helper's emotional energies, requiring on occasion understanding and support from colleagues. Perhaps it is no wonder, therefore, that bereavement is still to some extent a 'Cinderella' support service, and even specialist nurses, such as Macmillan home care teams have been found to put bereavement follow-up low if not bottom of their list of priorities (Lunt and Yardley, 1987).

In this chapter we have looked at the many ways we may be able to help bereaved people to meet their own needs. These may mean helping directly, for example, bereavement visiting, or indirectly, for example, by setting up a self-help group or a service run by volunteers.

REFERENCES

Baly, M. E., Robottom, B. and Clark, J. M. (1987) *District Nursing* (2nd edition), Heinemann, London.

Hopson, Barry (1982) Transition: understanding and managing personal change. In Chapman, A. J. and Gale, A. (eds.) *Psychology and People: A Tutorial Text*, British Psychological Society/Macmillan Press, London and Basingstoke.

Hubley, John (1982) Making the community profile. *Journal of the Institute of Health Education*, Vol. 20 (1).

Lunt, B. and Yardley, J. (1987) *A survey of home care teams and hospital support teams for the terminally ill*, unpublished report, National Society for Cancer Relief.

Osterweis, M., Soloman, F. and Green, S. (eds) (1985) *Bereavement: Reactions, Consequences and Care*, Wiley and Sons, Chichester.

Parkes, C. M. (1970) The first year of bereavement: a longitudinal study of the reaction of London widows to the death of their husbands. *Psychiatry*, Vol. 33, p. 44.

Parkes, C. M. and Parkes, J. (1984) Hospital versus hospice care – re-evaluation after 10 years as seen by surviving spouses. *Postgraduate Medical Journal*, Vol. 60, pp. 120-4.

Parkes, C. M. (1980) Bereavement counselling and does it work? *British Medical Journal*, Vol. 281, pp. 3-6, 5 July.

Rapoport, L. (1970) Crisis intervention as a mode of treatment. In Roberts, R. W. and Nee, R. H. (eds.) *Theories of Social Casework*, University of Chicago Press, Chicago.

Robinson, Kate (1983) What is health? In Henderson, J. and Clark, J. (eds.) *Community Health*, Churchill Livingstone, London.

Vachon, M. L. S. *et al.* (1980) A controlled study of self-help intervention for widows. *American Journal of Psychiatry*, pp. 1384-6.

10. How Can We Help? – The Skills of Communication

What you are speaks so loudly, that I cannot hear what you say to the contrary.

Ralph Waldo Emerson (1803–82)

INTRODUCTION

After the death and the funeral are over, family and friends inevitably begin to withdraw some of their support and practical help. Often they feel very guilty about this and have some awkwardness in deciding when and in what way they can do it. Their own needs and responsibility have often taken second place for some time and the bereaved person may have come to rely on them, particularly where there has been a long illness. When meeting them in the role of bereavement visitor, they are invariable defensive and apologetic, and these guilty feelings appear to be a direct result of the lack of prescribed ritual surrounding mourning. Comments such as 'I feel awful about it but I've got to go home sometime', 'I'm afraid he'll expect me to come down every weekend if I don't stop it soon'. 'I can't go on ringing up every evening, it's expensive for one thing and it's a tie', 'He's going to have to learn to cook for himself eventually', or 'My husband has been very understanding but he needs me too', demonstrate an apparent conflict between what many people *want* to do and what they feel they *should* do during the initial period of mourning that follows the funeral.

When someone we know has been bereaved, whether they are family or friend, colleague or a patient's relative, our natural reaction is to want to help them in some way. This sounds simple enough, yet I have found, and you may have done too, that in practice feelings of awkwardness and diffidence may get in the way. We want to help but we are afraid of making them feel worse, of saying or doing the wrong thing.

The following list of statements (Table 10.1) are for you to consider, either by yourself or with a friend for comparison. They also make a starting point to any discussion on bereavement.

Table 10.1 Bereavement 'quiz'. From *The Good Health Guide* (Open University), Pan Books (1982), with permission

If a friend were bereaved, I would	You	Friend or partner
accept their behaviour no matter how odd		
ignore their loss, pretend it never happened		
tell them about all my own woes		
let them cry and talk as much as they want		
tell them they are luckier than some		
give plenty of sympathy		
leave them well alone		
help them with practical problems		
tell them about everyone else's misfortunes		
take some burden of everyday chores away		
tell them they'll get over it eventually		
provide food and encourage sleep		
talk about the weather		
try to make them laugh		
stick around for when I'm needed		
tell them it could have been worse		
leave them out of my social circle		
tell them not to worry or think about it		
encourage them to go to the doctor for tablets		

STATEMENTS ON BEREAVEMENT

If a friend were bereaved, I would:

'accept their behaviour no matter how odd'

This is easy to write but not so easy to put into practice. You may feel that it depends on what the behaviour is. We also have a responsibility to that person to inform their general practitioner if we feel that their behaviour makes them at risk in any way.

'ignore their loss, pretend it never happened'

This is a common approach apparently adopted to protect the bereaved person yet, of course, at the same time protecting the helper. It is also a reflection of the desire not to intrude in any way (a very British approach, do you not think?). As we have seen, this is usually the last thing the bereaved person wants. They wish to have their loss acknowledged and respected.

'tell them about all my own woes'

This is a vain attempt to make the bereaved person feel better by reminding them that others have problems which may be worse. Statements such as 'I do understand' or 'I know how you feel' can make the bereaved person feel more isolated because they know that no-one else can fully understand their anguish at that time.

'let them cry and talk as much as they want'

As we have seen, this can be helpful in the appropriate situation as long as we are sure beforehand that we have the time and the energy to give and that we can help them to get themselves together again before we leave them. It may also be salutary to remember the study by Freihofer and Felton (see Chapter 4, page 50) which showed that relatives did not want to be encouraged to express their emotions before the death.

'tell them they are luckier than some'

This is another vain attempt to make the bereaved person feel better, this time by reminding them of all they have to be happy about. In their own time, the bereaved person may well be able to take comfort in their blessings but it can be very hurtful to receive this approach from others. This situation is exemplified by the classic statements often made to women who have lost children, 'You can always have another one!' or 'You've got the other children, which is more than many women have got'.

'give plenty of sympathy'

At first glance you probably agree that this is appropriate. A word more often used in the kind of context is *empathy*, conveying the idea that one is trying to enter into the other person's experience. Both need some caution in their use for they can be somewhat belittling, taking dignity away from the bereaved person. Respect for them and their feelings is probably what we are aiming for.

'leave them well alone'

Sometimes this is very appropriate. It is comforting when family and friends rally round but too much attention and company can be tiring. The bereaved person may feel that they need some time to themselves, to cry and to think. 'I wanted to have some time in my house on my own, when my baby died,' said one woman, 'in order to think through all that had happened and make sense of it. I also preferred to express my feelings on my own on some occasions.'

'help them with practical problems'

This is usually a very much appreciated way of showing the bereaved person that you care about them. At first, some practical problems can seem insurmountable. What this should not mean is that the carer takes over. For example, I found it very helpful when a friend took me out for the first time to do some Christmas shopping. I was also helped by a large number of friends who took my children to and from school until

I was able to do it myself. The friend who left pies and cakes on the front door step was also helping practically with feeding the family, and also showing much thought and concern.

'tell them about everyone else's misfortunes'

Like telling the bereaved about your own problems, this is not helpful. The bereaved person will gradually and in their own way become aware of what they share with others who have had devastating problems.

'take some burden of everyday chores away'

This can be very helpful at the beginning, in particular taking over some of the chores usually done by the person who has died. It may be useful to show the bereaved person how to do these themselves, a good example being to help the bereaved husband to cook for himself or the bereaved wife how to light the boiler. It can be therapeutic for children in the family to be shown how to do these sort of jobs so that they feel they are helping.

'tell them they'll get over it eventually'

If done with sensitivity to what the bereaved person is saying, it can be encouraging to hear that others have been through a similar experience and felt in a similar way, and have come through it. This is the base for the success of self-help groups. It is only effective if you are able to tell them truthfully that either you or someone you have known has come to terms with a similar bereavement experience.

'provide food and encourage sleep'

This can be associated with the earlier discussion concerning the general physical health of the bereaved person and its link with coping with major stress. Sometimes a fitness regime can be a positive help at an appropriate stage.

'talk about the weather'

This indicates the need in the carer to divert the bereaved person from their pain and it may often be a vain attempt. However, we must also remember that social chitchat also meets a need for normality and security, and people going through an emotional crisis do not always and at all times want to talk about it. A balance is what we try to aim for.

'try to make them laugh'

It is inappropriate to say to a grieving person 'give us a smile!' when they patently do not feel like it. On the other hand, just as laughter is closely related to tears it is possible to see that many sad situations have elements of laughter in them. It is part of life.

However, a bereaved person may feel much guilt at having enjoyed a joke or an amusing incident, and it can only be done spontaneously with sensitivity to their feelings.

'stick around for when I'm needed'

It is important to continue to offer whatever help you can, long after you think it may no longer be needed. We all rally round at first and, as we have seen, the newly bereaved person may refuse all offers of help, wanting to show to themselves as well as to others that they can cope. Days, weeks or even months later they may want some help and are very likely to want to talk about the deceased when others think they should not still wish to.

'tell them it could have been worse'

This is completely inappropriate statement in the circumstances. The loss of someone you love and are close to is the worst loss that can happen to any of us, so this kind of comment is irrelevant.

'leave them out of my social circle'

This is a common experience for bereaved people, especially women on their own. It is very unkind and creates another burden to bear. It says that they are not valued as individuals and that they are stigmatized. It is important to keep social contacts the same as before or to include people you know are now on their own.

'tell them not to worry or think about it'

This kind of statement is facile and conveys that the carer does not understand their needs at all.

'encourage them to go to their doctor for tablets'

Medication of any kind can only be useful *in the short-term* and is better avoided when possible. As we have seen, attempts to short-circuit the pain of mourning is not helpful to long-term adjustment. But it is often therapeutic to encourage a newly bereaved person to see their general practitioner so that potential health problems can be prevented or treated early on. Bereaved people with supportive family doctors find this adds to their feelings of security and provides long-term help.

For many bereaved people it is at this time that they begin to be left alone to come to terms with their loss and to find new ways of living. If some kind of support or follow-up could be provided, then this would seem to be the appropriate time for it to be offered.

In visiting a bereaved person the nurse has, I suggest, two main roles: assessor and counsellor. The first decision she has to make is *when* to visit. The aim, of course, is to visit when family and friends have begun to withdraw their support, approximately four to six weeks after the death. If further visits are appropriate, then it is often possible to negotiate with the bereaved person themselves as to when they might find this helpful. Anniversaries of all kinds are times when a bereaved person may feel particularly vulnerable. 'I'd like you to come the middle of next month because it's our wedding anniversary,' is the kind of comment often made.

It is often helpful to visit, telephone, or send a personal card or note on the anniversary of the death of the patient. The decision to do this depends on the perceived need, or the relationship between the helper and bereaved person, and on the other commitments the helper has.

The following guidelines for helpers are not intended to be a blueprint, or to be rigidly followed. My colleagues and I found them helpful, especially in the early stages, as a means of concentrating mind and energy prior to the visit and as a useful tool for reflecting on it and writing it up afterwards.

BEREAVEMENT VISITS: GUIDELINES FOR HELPERS

Name of deceased person   Age
When they died
Where death took place
Their relationship to key person

Key person
Address   Tel. no.

Occupation (including voluntary work etc)

Family
Children (list all names, ages and locations)

Other living relatives and/or very close friends

General comments

Home and Environment
Type, others living there, space, any problems

Key person's attitude to visit
Welcomed/strongly welcomed/accepted/accepted reluctantly/refused
If reluctant or refused, what happened?

Need for support
Very great/great/moderate/some/none/probably harmful

Observations (checklist)
Appearance: well-groomed/casual but tidy/untidy/dirty and unkempt
Activity: slow/normal/some agitation and jumpiness/restlessness
Tearfulness: continuous tears/frequent/some/suppressed/no sign
Very sad/sad/variable sadness/neutral/happy/elated
Severe anxiety/some anxiety/neutral/calm/very calm
Risk of possible suicide: immediate/likely/remote/unlikely/none
Very angry over many things/angry over few things/minor irritability or
   anger/no evidence of anger/denies anger or irritability
Targets of anger
Preoccupations: intense guilt/marked guilt or self-approach/some minor
   self-reproach/no evidence/denied

Potential problems (as identified by the bereaved person)
No problems
Lack of contact with others, isolation and loneliness
Excessive crying
Eating too much or too little
Sleeping badly
Smoking too much
Drinking too much alcohol
Medication: too much/not enough
Illness: actual physical illness/fear of physical illness
Fears of having a 'breakdown', 'going mad' or haunting memories
Job: wanting a job/coping with a job/wanting to give up a job
Money: managing money/insufficient money for needs
Accommodation: getting accommodation/keeping existing home/man-
   aging housework
Death: seeking to explain or understand the death
God: doubts concerning goodness of God/doubts concerning *afterlife*/
   concerning existence of God
Belief: other spiritual or religious problems/doubts concerning own
   goodness or worth/doubts about goodness or worth of others
Relationships: difficult in maintaining relationships with family/friends/
   difficulty in coping with children's grief/difficulty in explaining death
   to children/difficulty in controlling children's behaviour

Help offered or given
None
Opportunity to talk through feelings, problems
Specific advice
Direct help
Referral to other help: minister/social worker/health visitor/doctor/ general practitioner/other/nurse/volunteer
Housing department/social security/social services/solicitor/citizens advice bureau/Samaritans/self-help organizations/occupational health department/school teacher

---

Probably the most useful sense when assessing others is one's 'sixth sense', or intuition. This is, after all, born of experience and should prompt us to seek help and advice even when other signs of problems seem to be missing. We need to remember that the person at home is under the care of their general practitioner and our responsibility is to report to him or her any concerns we have about them.

Counselling

This term is used to describe the use of various techniques to help people to adjust to a changed social environment, so it is a concept that can readily be applied to trying to help the bereaved person. It is defined in The Ethics of the British Association for Counselling (1984) as 'giving the client an opportunity to explore, discover and clarify ways of living more satisfyingly and resourcefully'. Its main features are that communication is always a two-way process, it is non-judgemental in approach and it focuses on problems identified by clients themselves, with implicit ideas of personal fulfilment and growth.

The other essential role of the helper is that of counsellor. Counselling has become a jargon word much overused in professional circles. Sometimes it would seem to include almost any one-to-one communication and, in nursing, it can even be used to describe disciplinary activities! The use of the word to define a role ranging from beauty counsellor to investment counsellor or from marriage guidance counsellor to abortion counsellor means that it has become a loose term, rather mysterious and 'special'.

There are many different models of counselling. As nurses we are familiar with the nursing process and, therefore, the Wessex Model of

Counselling (Stewart, 1983) provides a useful starting point as its stages correspond to those of the nursing process (Figure 10.1 and 10.2). It is a systematic approach to counselling, helping the nurse to structure her thinking, but in use it can be both flexible and dynamic.

Figure 10.1 Wessex model of counselling. Source: Stewart, W. (1983) *Counselling in Nursing: A Problem-solving Approach* (Lippincott Nursing Series), with kind permission

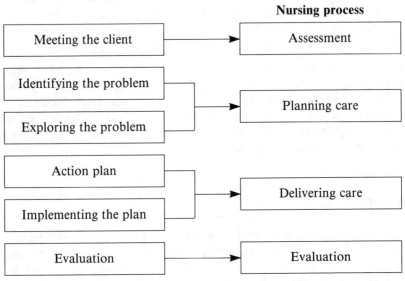

Figure 10.2

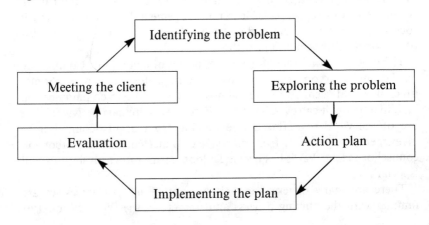

THE BEREAVEMENT VISIT

David Stoater (1987) sees the initial task as being to make the person feel comfortable to have you with them. The interpersonal skills needed to do this are ones that should be taught and practised by all nurses as they are essential to nursing practice.

In order to be able to enter into a helping relationship with a bereaved person, it appears necessary to have an awareness of one's own reactions to loss and to have thought through, to some extent at least, one's attitude to death – which means of course one's attitude to life itself. Speck (1978) points this out and adds that the professional helper may well face particular problems in finding the 'courage and the confidence to remain human'.

This I have certainly found to be true. It is naturally tempting to maintain distance from a distressed person if one feels inadequate and afraid, by trying to hide behind the professional role.

What the helper is trying to do is to give, in a sense, permission to the bereaved person to express how they feel, which includes many uncomfortable emotions. The helper is there to assist them in reviewing the relationship with all its positive and negative aspects, and sometimes other losses will be brought out at this time, usually because they have not been resolved previously.

Therefore, the main tasks are to provide a caring environment where the bereaved person feels able to talk if they so wish, to reassure them of the normality of the strong emotions that are being expressed and then, when possible, to help point towards a realistic and positive adjustment to the new pattern of life.

The importance is in sharing the burden but not becoming involved, giving in to one's own feelings and therefore losing perspective of the supporting role.

This balance is, as you may have experienced, hard to maintain – to find one's own appropriate place emotionally.

Weiss and Parkes (1981) found that the central problem when working with bereaved people was not in initiating the expression of grief but, more importantly, in terminating it. They suggest that it is possible for helpers to inadvertently collude in perpetuating grief. When planning to visit a bereaved person, the helper must allow adequate time. It must always be borne in mind that the bereaved person may not decide to talk about how they feel until the apparent end of the visit. Many times I have made a social visit discussing everything from the current political scene to pruning roses, only to have my hand on the door knob or the latch of the front gate when the bereaved person has trusted me sufficiently to begin to talk about how things really are for them.

Immediately prior to the visit, especially when you are inexperienced and feeling understandably apprehensive, it is helpful to take five minutes, perhaps parked round the corner, to breathe deeply and relax so that you do not feel rushed. Try to clear the mind of all the other tasks and reponsibilities of the day. This will help you to concentrate on the verbal and non-verbal aspects of the communication and to avoid clumsiness such as rapid talking or sitting in a tense position. One of the most difficult skills I had to learn, and I know many nurses have found this too, was to feel comfortable with silence. I found it hard to allow the bereaved person time to collect their thoughts, without experiencing an overwhelming desire to fill the space!

It is not always possible, in someone else's home, to choose where to sit. Sitting directly opposite the bereaved person can appear very suitable for a professional interview, but it may make the bereaved person feel uncomfortable without knowing why. It is the position of confrontation and tends to give the impression that the helper is the one who is in charge. Standing, particularly when the helper is taller than the clients, can also give this impression.

We have mentioned the skill of active listening and it is undoubtedly important to concentrate carefully on all that may be said to us, yet it is possible to overdo this too. Too much attention can be felt as an intrusion, the helper can appear very intense and this makes the bereaved person feel defensive.

One of the best positions in my experience is to sit at the side of the bereaved person. This means they can most easily look away and avoid the helper when they feel like it and it tends to convey a feeling that both people are looking at the situation from a similar perspective. Much is talked about the value of physical contact during such an interview and, when used appropriately, it can change the nature of it considerably. However, sensitivity is needed here.

Culturally, we British are not 'touchers' and inappropriate touching can imply an intimacy that the bereaved person may not like, particularly when reflecting on the encounter later. Much may depend on whether there has been a relationship with the bereaved person previously, or whether a new one is being established.

The interview should be, as far as is possible, judgement-free. This may sound obvious, yet if we think more deeply we begin to realize how difficult it is to put on one side opinions and attitudes that have been built up during our lifetime. One aim is to receive and affirm whatever the bereaved person may choose to tell us, which involves us being as open and responsive as we can and to respect their honesty. For them to be honest, particularly about negative, uncomfortable feelings or relationship breakdowns, takes courage and is about letting go of whatever they may feel, and this may have been there for a very long time. As a helper you have to consider whether you really do want them to do this with you. If you think of encounters with small children and how uncomfortable these can sometimes be, you may decide that it is very hard to live within the limits of honesty. Encouraging that honesty means accepting how this may make you feel, and also considering whether you have sufficient time for this to happen.

However open and non-judgemental the helper may feel, it is still easy to come to hasty conclusions about what the bereaved person may be trying to explain – both to you and to themselves. This may not be a correct interpretation, so the aim must be to put oneself, as far as possible, to one side and try to hear what the bereaved person is trying to say, both verbally or non-verbally. Being honest and genuine is very important; as Emerson said, 'What you are speaks so loudly that I cannot hear what you say to the contrary'.

As I discussed earlier, many of us find silence uncomfortable. Practising relaxation techniques such as concentrating on breathing can be useful as these cause the helper to relax and feel comfortable, allowing the bereaved person the time to put difficult thoughts into words, to open up what is in them. When we are in deep trouble, we tend to regress somewhat towards childhood, and emotions and expressions of feeling seem to become more childlike. The bereaved person is looking, therefore, for some warmth and comfort from the helper.

Many bereaved people want to express feelings of guilt. Sometimes, of course, there are grounds for feeling guilty but often there appears to be none. In either case, reassurance is being looked for, although I have found that its value is limited – for example, the wife who found her husband in the garden having suffered a heart attack, and who tried with neighbours to resuscitate him but failed. It may be of some value to be able to say 'You gave him a chance! You were not able to succeed, but this was *not* your fault!' Equally important is to allow this lady to explore how she feels about it and to tell the helper 'her story' of what happened.

When talking with students and trained nurses about helping people in distress or in a crisis situation, I have always found that a major concern is what the helper should actually say in any given situation. Yet the more experience we have it seems the less we need to be concerned about the actual words we use, as long as they are the expression of honest caring and feeling towards that person we are trying to help. There are, of course, some stock phrases which are usually better avoided and usually reflect a lack of forethought or understanding of the situation.

For example, it is rarely useful to say to a bereaved person, 'I understand how you feel', even if you have been bereaved yourself. Each relationship and loss is unique for each individual and what you are really doing is bolstering up your own ego rather than saying anything of use to the bereaved person. If they turn to you, the helper, and say that you seem to understand, that is different because it has come from them, not you.

Another common example is provided by the bereaved person who, in the helper's opinion, seems to be doing remarkably well, but is explaining how vulnerable, incompetent and useless they are feeling. The tempting retort is 'But you are coping so well!' This may seem like worthwhile encouragement, but what it does is to block out what they are feeling and take away any chance of telling us that they are not coping as well as everyone thinks.

So if we take on the role of helper to a bereaved person, what are we trying to do? What outcomes are we intending? Are these likely to be the same or different from what the bereaved person is hoping for?

The skills of active listening, the use of open and closed questioning, how to respond to difficult behaviour and different ways of intervening are all core skills, the teaching of which are beyond the scope of this book. If you feel that you have not been taught these adequately or that you have not had sufficient practice or that there is (always!) room for improvement, please turn to the suggested reading list at the end of the chapter (for example, Kagan, Evans and Kay, 1986; Burnard, 1985; Tschudin, 1987; Bond, 1986, etc.) A lot can be achieved by reading and then trying out the exercises and suggestions made there, and then evaluating both the outcome and the process that led to it.

TOOLS FOR HELPING

It may be useful to underline one facet of the philosophy of a helping relationship: whatever is offered to the client it has to be a free gift! Yet, it is tempting when with a distressed and potentially grateful bereaved person to promise more than we are able to give. That is, it is made without reservation, qualifications or a profit and loss account. The helper is not there to cost the bereaved person energy, not to make them feel grateful or subservient in any way. The resource and time available has no strings attached. Neither does the helping relationship allow for the helper to become a prop of any kind, because this is about meeting possible needs in the helper, not in the client. A long-term goal must be independence and the strength that comes from relying on one's own resources.

It has been suggested that in order to be able to do this the helper acts like a pair of jump leads, providing the energy to get the 'bereaved car' started. The helper needs to have the spare resource to do this. This often means that they too need support from others. Yet professional people tend not to ask or expect this, sometimes seeing the need for it as meaning that they are lacking in some way, an admittance of not coping. This has often been the case in nursing.

Yet, attempting to help bereaved and other distressed people means that fundamentally we have to accept that we are all *potentially* non-copers, that both you or I could be at risk during bereavement. We are potential suicides, alcoholics, drug addicts, difficult teenagers, etc. We may have been any of these in the past. In other words, we are all capable of losing control and to be angry and bewildered if we lose it. Acceptance of this fact is necessary, I suggest, in order to provide a supportive service for bereaved people, We are not 'experts'. We are all ultimately dependent on each other.

COMMUNICATION

The preparation, team support and communication skills that are necessary for nurses to be able to support relatives are, of course, also needed when caring for families before death. Professional attitudes to death may be to do with a sense of failure, both of ourselves and of medical science. Feelings of inadequacy and a lack of control may make nurses feel ill-prepared and unsupported.

Caring for bereaved families and dying patients present many difficulties for medical and nursing staff; Maguire and Faulkner (1988) suggest that these ought to be acknowledged more openly and dealt with more adequately, because the emotional price may sometimes be too high for the individual. Perhaps we, as members of society, expect too much.

Staff learn to distance themselves from their patients as an effective defence mechanism. They ignore cues about emotionally loaded areas by such techniques as:

- jollying along: 'there's no need to look so glum, the sun is shining!'
- premature reassurance: 'You're bound to be upset that you've still got a lot of pain – but we'll up your pain killers.'
- false reassurance: 'I'm sure your sickness will get better – we've got good antiemetics these days.'

- normalizations: 'Everybody feels upset when they first come in here but you'll soon get used to it.'
- switching tactics: (patient) 'I can't understand why I've lost so much weight', (nurse) 'Have you had any trouble with your bowels?'
- passing the buck: (patient) 'Am I getting better? (nurse), 'You'll have to ask the doctor that one,'; or (patient) 'I've been very upset', (nurse) 'I'll ask the social worker to come and see you.'

Few of us have not been guilty of using some of these tactics.

When Maguire and Faulkner (1988) carried out a series of studies to determine the extent to which patients failed to cope with uncertainty of prognosis and treatment they found that between one-quarter and one-third of patients and families developed an anxiety state or depressive illness. They also found that little of this psychiatric morbidity was disclosed by the patient or recognized by the doctors, nurses and social workers. Generally, 80 per cent remained unrecognized and untreated, pointing perhaps to avoidance strategies being practised by the professional staff involved.

Distance is not likely to be due to a lack of concern but may be adopted to help the individual survive emotionally; becoming close to patients means that each death may be experienced as a loss by the nurse.

Getting close to distressed relatives reminds us of our own losses; it may cause us to question our views of life and death and our caring abilities. It is easier, for example, not to become the patient or family's advocate and, for example, question chemotherapy for a dying patient or ask for more analgesia for a patient on their own and/or the family's behalf. This causes us to concentrate on practical problems that are likely to be resolved.

There is danger they may become stressed and suffer what Americans refer to as 'burn out'. Health is adversely affected and physical complaints such as exhaustion, insomnia and minor illnesses, and irritability, withdrawal from socializing, rigidity of outlook and, finally, withdrawal from work with feelings of guilt may be experienced.

Effective and appropriate training on communication and counselling skills to be able to help bereaved people effectively but safely from their own standpoint are needed, and workshops are one way of providing this kind of education.

This chapter has looked at the skills needed to be able to offer help to bereaved people who may be met by professionals and by volunteers. Whether you are a hospital or community care nurse, a Macmillan health visitor, specialist nurse community psychiatric nurse or midwife, the role is essentially that of a facilitator. It is often that of an innovator as well, promoting initiative within the community.

REFERENCES

Bond, Meg (1986) *Stress and Self Awareness: A Guide for Nurses*, Heineman, London.

British Association for Counselling (1984) *Code of Ethics*, 1:2.

Burnard, Philip (1985) *Learning Human Skills: A Guide for Nurses*, Heineman, London.

The Good Health Guide (1982) Open University, Pan Books, London.

Kagan, C., Evans, J. and Kay, B. (1986) *A Manual of Interpersonal Skills for Nurses. An Experimental Approach* (Lippincott Nursing Series), Harper and Row, London.

Maguire, Peter and Faulkner, Ann (1988) Communicate with cancer patients: handling uncertainty, collusion and denial, *British Medical Journal*, Vol. 297, pp. 972–4.

Parkes, C. M. and Weiss, R. S. (1981) *Recovery from Bereavement*, Basic Books Inc., New York.

Speck, Peter (1978) *Loss and Grief in Medicine*, Baillière Tindall, London.

Stewart, William (1983) *Counselling in Nursing: A Problem-Solving Approach* (Lippincott Nursing Series), Harper and Row, London.

Stoater, David (1987) Paper presented at the Palliative Care for European Nurses Seminar at Napp Laboratories, Cambridge.

Tschudin, Verena (1987) *Counselling Skills for Nurses*, Baillière Tindall, London.

Webster, Margaret E. (1981) Communicating with dying patients. *Nursing Times*, Vol. 77(23), pp. 999–1002.

11. The Way Forward: Selection, Support and Education for Nurses

Education is an admirable thing, but it is well to remember from time to time that nothing that is worth knowing can be taught.

Oscar Wilde (1854–1900)

INTRODUCTION

As we have seen, the experience of being bereaved is as old as life – and death – itself. Whether it is discussed in terms of attachment and separation (Bowlby, 1981), a process (Parkes, 1972) or as a series of tasks (Worden, 1984) or as a life transition (Hopson and Scally, 1979), it is a natural phenomenon. Therefore, the first question to be asked is how much education, if any, is needed?

It was the philosopher Illich (1976) who first alerted us to the possible dangers of what he called the medicalization of life events. By this he meant that events such as birth and death are often taken over by the medical and health care professions, power and control being taken away from the individual. Is there a danger that we have overstressed the significance of bereavement in terms of mortality and morbidity and, if we provide various kinds of bereavement support services, begin to treat it as an illness?

It is part of the philosophy of our times that our health and wellbeing are considered to be our own responsibility. So, when we are bereaved should we not be able to deal effectively with our predicament, drawing on coping skills we have used in the past? Should there be any need for outside interventions of any kind?

Is not bereavement support simply common sense? Does it require only a 'tender loving care' approach? If the helper has also been bereaved, does this constitute sufficient preparation for helping others? If the helper means well will all be well? Not necessarily, I suggest. A lack of knowledge and skills can make the helper feel inadequate and helpless. A lack of self-awareness may cause them to be over-protective or over-sentimental in their approach. It is unlikely that any of us can be taught to care but it is possible to teach us to be more effective in that caring.

STAFF SELECTION

Staff selection, whether professional or volunteer is always a difficult area. When working with bereaved people it is particularly important to find out why the individual wants to do this. A previous loss that has not yet been resolved may prompt an individual to offer help which they may not yet have the energy to give. This may be the death of a loved friend or relative but it could also be recent divorce, broken engagement or loss of expected promotion. Guidance towards a self-help group may be appropriate.

An individual with very strong beliefs or prejudices may feel superior and all-powerful in the role of helper and view the bereaved person as helpless. If they have rigid ideas of a religious nature they may want to convert those they visit, and find it hard to accept views that are very different. They also need to be directed towards other ways of helping people.

The likely compatibility of the individual with other team members is always a concern when selecting staff. The person who is practical and has a positive approach to life, who fits in and makes others feel comfortable to have them there, has traits that can obviously be utilized in any kind of supportive service.

Tschudin (1985) identified four broad areas for consideration when planning staff support systems:

- education and training;
- occupational health departments;
- counselling services;
- support groups.

Education and training

So what is there to teach? The answer to this question must be based on the objectives that have been agreed for the particular bereavement support service. Although there are likely to be some variations, it would appear that the helper has two main functions: assessment and counselling. Both of these require appropriate knowledge, attitudes and skills. What knowledge is needed by someone who has *already* experienced bereavement? What level of information might be necessary for someone who has not done so?

Everyone has experienced some kind of loss in their lives. Therefore, an obvious starting point is to assess the existing knowledge of loss and bereavement present in any group and to begin by building on that. In this way, the acquisition of knowledge proceeds from the known to the unknown. Most people, in my experience, know more than they think they do! It is also valuable to adopt this approach in order to build confidence. The knowledge gained should not be prescriptive but enhance the helper's assessment of those potentially at risk of complications during mourning.

When planning such teaching I find it useful to consider the intended results in terms of the first three of Bloom's (1956) categories of the cognitive domain. This is the area of learning concerned with intellectual outcomes.

(1) **Knowledge**: simple knowledge of facts, of terms and of theories; this would be likely to include different perspectives on loss and bereavement, a consideration of at risk groups and current research.

(2) **Comprehension**: an understanding of the meaning of this knowledge; this can be tested out by questioning and discussion.

(3) **Application**: the ability to apply this knowledge and comprehension in new and concrete situations; information can be illustrated with examples from practice and the helpers asked to make links with their own experience.

Attitudes are the next component for consideration. They are not, of course, totally separate from knowledge, indeed the values and expectations that the individual holds will colour that knowledge and may affect what he chooses to remember. Kalish suggests that the behaviours surrounding death and bereavement are among the cultural features that are the 'most conservative and most resistant to change'.

Ideas of what is usual or unusual behaviour before, at the time of, or after the death and how this is interpreted is knowledge involving beliefs.

They are derived from the earliest socialization and reinforced or altered by the social group in which the individual now belongs. They are both descriptive and explanatory.

Therefore, the attitudes of the helpers also need to be explored early on. Here my planning would take account of the effective domain (of Krathwohl *et al.*, 1964).

(1) **Receiving**: this refers to the willingness to attend or listen, the motivation of the individual is also involved; however, the helper may be motivated to help but not think they have anything to learn.
(2) **Responding**: this is the willingness to participate; this is not only about active involvement but includes the quiet, thoughtful helper who is involved in what is going on but lacks the confidence to participate directly.
(3) **Valuing**: this involves the exploration of the individual's personal belief system on which their decisions may be based.
(4) **Organizing**: this level may also be applicable where the helper, through increased self-knowledge and openness to different ideas and viewpoints, may actually modify some of the attitudes and opinions with which they started out.

The acquisition of skills comes from relating knowledge to practice and by learning and using a wide range of interpersonal skills. This is preparation for the role of counsellor, a very overworked word and often used loosely. I sometimes feel it is impossible to have any communication on a one-to-one basis without labelling it as 'counselling'! However, its main features are that any interaction is always a two-way process, its approach is non-judgemental and its focus is on client-centred problems. This last point is particularly important. It means practice in putting one's own perception on one side and to be actively involved with the bereaved person's concerns – which may well be different from the helper's expectations. A starting point here is the widening of personal experience through increased self-awareness and self-knowledge.

The very word 'education' is derived from *educare*, Latin for 'to bring out that which is already there'. Therefore, it is important to recognize that people bring to the role of helper everything that they are. Many will be volunteers and their contribution in terms of maturity and life experiences must never be underestimated.

How we teach is intimately linked with how we learn. Research supports the view that most learning takes place by active participation, that is by exploring, imitating and *doing*. One of the most effective methods, widely recognized in specialist medical education, is to work with an experienced person. After all, teaching is not confined to professional teachers and learners; wherever the inexperienced and those with expertise are together some kind of learning is going on.

However the needs of the learner have to be balanced against the needs of the bereaved person. Having an extra person present, no matter how discreet, inevitably alters the interaction between the helper and the bereaved person, whether in a negative or positive way. My own experience of taking learners with me on visits to bereaved people was rarely problematic, leading me to question my initial reservations, which may have been based on my own insecurities rather than on evidence of interference with what I was hoping to do.

However, even when it is possible to provide experience 'on the job' it is still necessary, I suggest, to make provision for some learning to take place outside of bereavement visits or groups.

Bearing in mind Tyler's (1949) guiding principle that no *single* learning experience has a very profound influence upon the learner, a variety of methods can and should be used. These are intended to provide opportunities for the individual to explore their experiences and feelings. Bruner (1966) alerts us to the potential problem inherent in these kind of approaches; that their adoption can become 'an excuse for vague and haphazard goings-on'. Therefore it is important that sessions are planned beforehand and are structured.

Attention to the available environment is an important initial consideration. We all have ideas of what would constitute ideal surroundings, construction and size of the group, but reality may dictate something quite different! I have run various workshops for professional and volunteer helpers in such diverse situations as the local library, church and village halls, hotel and conference room, hotel ballroom, classrooms both in colleges and schools of nursing, in an individual's own home and in a church! Group size has ranged from 12 to 50 +. Flexibility is obviously essential and making the best of what you have means creating as relaxed and informal an atmosphere as you can.

Formal lectures are rarely appropriate. Short talks to provide information followed by questions and discussions are, I find, useful ways of beginning to work and encouraging participation in a non-threatening way. It is important to value each contribution but, at the same time, to guide the group so that the main objectives of the session can be achieved.

Case studies, starting with straightforward situations and progressing to ones that illustrate typical problems are invaluable ways of relating knowledge gained to what is likely to be encountered by the new helper.

Working in pairs and/or small groups and then feeding back ideas to the main group invariably produces lively exchanges which, once again, need to be tactfully and unobtrusively managed.

Workshops are an effective way of practising skills. There needs to be plenty of time to build confidence and group cohesion and to allow for self-consciousness at the beginning. I find it helpful to ask the group, at the start, for their ideas of what is going to happen so that their expect-ations and anxieties can be expressed and shared. Burnard (1985), des-cribing a workshop exploring methods of coping with emotional release (obviously an essential topic area for those involved in bereavement work), points out that when other people become emotionally upset, we often become distressed ourselves. If even only one participant appears to be in difficulty, embarrassment and confusion can quickly run through the others. Once again, careful and sensitive management is essential.

Role-play is a high profile method for all kinds of work in the interpersonal skills area. However, I approach it with great caution. I would never use it where I did not know the group over a period of time or where the group members did not know each other well and were not very cohesive. In any group there may be members who have recently been bereaved or have 'hidden' bereavements (abortion or miscarriage for example, or simply a loss they have not acknowledged to the group). There may be unresolved bereavements or losses in their past (loss through an earlier divorce, for example, or a childhood bereavement that has never been worked through). In other words, role-play can be a minefield. However, when used appropriately with supportive small groups it is a very effective way of exploring feelings and practising skills. Role-reversal can be particularly useful in providing insights into the experiences and perceptions of others. It is very important that adequate time is left at the end of such a session for a full 'processing' of the experience.

Reinforcement is an important learning principle. It can be useful and illuminating to bring a group of helpers back together again after a period of providing bereavement support. This serves both as refresh-ment for them, being a chance to review past and present learning and to share new ideas, and as reinforcement of the knowledge and attitudes originally taught. It is also a way for them to support each other. It can be helpful to the teacher as it offers an opportunity to evaluate teaching in terms of both process and product.

Tyler's model of teaching and learning provides a summary of these points. The four questions he asks are:

(1) What is the purpose of the teaching situation? (Aims)
(2) What experiences can we provide? (Content)
(3) How can these be organized? (Method and organization)
(4) How do we know that these experiences have been useful? (Evaluation)

Number 4 is, of course, the 'crunch question'. Is this kind of learning measurable? We cannot objectively measure it but, I suggest, by developing intuition – which is, after all, knowledge borne of experience – the helper may be able to evaluate the process that went on between them and the bereaved person. What may or may not have been prevented in terms of morbidity or mortality, let alone straightforward human unhappiness, is inevitably hard to quantify.

In all this it can be seen that the teacher's role may encompass that of group leader, manager and facilitator rather than as a purveyor of knowledge who may appear to be remote from the individual's own experience.

During this brief look at what the field of education may have to offer helpers involved in bereavement support, I have not intended to suggest that it can equip them to meet every need, to relieve every situation. On the contrary, one of the myths that has to be dispelled early on is that the helper can actually help everyone. No-one can remove, or help the bereaved remove, all the obstacles in any individual's life. Common sense about human nature is needed, as is humanity about ourselves.

Neither is bereavement support all 'sweetness and light'. Relatives may hate the person who died (and feel very guilty about it). There may be complex family problems. Worse still, the bereaved person may not always appear grateful for the time and effort made by the helper; they may even occasionally hate them too!

We are all of course, teachers and learners, 'mentors' to other nurses. Much of our learning, both for good and ill, is 'taught' as we go through life. I suggest that what we are 'taught' is of equal value when attempting to support bereaved people. Bereavement is about death and, therefore, also about life and many helpers are drawn to this work because they are sorting out their personal philosophy. This is not new. Plato wrote, 'What matters most is *not* the knowledge imparted to a man but what the man himself becomes in the course of acquiring that knowledge'. I suspect that this is what much of education for bereavement support is really about.

The structure of work must be looked at so that staff are able to share with others, to spend time away from patients, as teachers, for example.

Perhaps a deliberate policy of a certain time limit for working in this field needs to be looked at. Sabbatical leave is one option used in America where staff working at Hospice Inc., Newhaven, Connecticut, can for example take additional annual leave compared with staff working in other medical, nursing or social work areas.

Occupational health departments

These exist both in industry and in the National Health Service and are mainly staffed by nurses, usually with part-time support from a doctor. Training for the Occupational Health Certificate is not yet mandatory, but consists of eighteen months' part-time or six months' full-time study.

Within the National Health Service, it is still difficult to get across to many nurses that occupational health nurses are not part of the management structure but are concerned with the individual and her needs in a confidential relationship. In many health authorities this independence is emphasized by the lack of titles or uniform of the occupational health nurses.

Their main functions are prevention of illness, health education and screening. They are also concerned with the effect of the working environment on the health of the individual.

They may also, from time to time, act as counsellors, providing first-line support and referring to more specialized help if and when this is needed. So at any time they may be concerned with the health of a worker who has been bereaved if this either directly or indirectly affects their work.

Counselling services

As long ago as 1972, the Briggs Committee on Nursing advocated a comprehensive counselling service for nurses working in all areas. It would be necessary for these to be independent of professional or bureaucratic organizations and to maintain confidentiality. Crawley (1984) recommends that health authorities should make counselling services available to all groups of staff. Co-counselling is often found to be useful by nurses, where two colleagues meet regularly to share problems with each other. This works if it is formalized and seen by both people to be a commitment.

Support groups

Interdisciplinary groups: I see support as being about the creation of a multiprofessional team of people who are working towards common goals and who meet regularly to discuss both positive and negative aspects of their work. A leader who is skilled and charismatic can be useful, especially at the beginning. Rotating leadership may be appropriate – or no leadership at all!

Teamwork takes time and has to be seen as being important or it can easily be subjugated for seemingly more important or pressing matters. Creating a team takes time, it does not happen overnight. Its growth may be facilitated by group meetings and informal social events from time to time where people can appear as individuals rather than 'wearing' their professional roles. Support groups of nurses only can also be valuable. Either way, basic aims need to be agreed and regular meetings organized. There needs to be a commitment to the group, and where the contributions of every person from volunteer to doctor, from student to social worker is valued and encouraged.

Comfort may be found in remembering that these natural emotions are commonly felt and understandable. Staff who have grown close to the patient and family very naturally suffer some of the reactions of the bereaved for they too have suffered a loss. This has to be borne in mind when they are involved in continued contact with a family who are bereaved. It may be difficult for the staff themselves to 'let go' of a relative. It is also possible to become 'burnt out' by too much involvement for too long, with distressed people. The nurse can suffer from 'compassion fatigue' and react by withdrawing or becoming irritable.

The preparation of nurses to deal with all aspects of dying patients and their families should begin at the elementary stage of training where the nurse should be introduced to the concept of ageing, death and bereavement. It must continue to develop actively within the practice setting whether this is a hospital ward or in the community.

Studies of four nursing schools by Birch (1983) presented a generally unsatisfactory picture of the teaching of nurses about death and bereavement. It showed that caring for dying bereaved people was one of the most anxiety-provoking situations experienced by student nurses. A survey by Field (1984) suggested that death and bereavement were topics which were now receiving attention by schools of nursing and, interestingly, at a level that favourably compares with that found in medical schools in the United Kingdom. More hours were devoted to such teaching in nursing schools than medical schools over a shorter course duration and a greater variety of teaching methods were used. The fact that these topics were dealt with in more detail in nursing schools is, I think, a natural reflection of the differences in time which would be spent with patients and relatives by the respective professions. Nurses are more accessible to relatives and they are more likely to feel able to ask questions than when making a specific appointment to see a doctor.

Caughill (1976) noted that nurses appear to suffer the same distress as everyone else when caring for the dying, since few seemed to be any better prepared than the lay person to deal with the realities of death. In a study conducted by Le Shan (1976), nurses felt inadequate in interacting with dying patients. He discovered that it took nurses significantly longer to respond to terminal patients than to other severely ill patients when they called for assistance.

Webster (1981) pointed out that nurses are not likely to have been encouraged to talk about death at any time in their lives. She goes on to say that 'it seems much more likely that they will have been socialized into the idea that death is something that you just do not talk about'. It seems unrealistic, therefore, to expect that they would suddenly shed all trace of this early socialization and start to accept death without some very specialized preparation.

Field and Kitson (1986) looked at schools of nursing and found that 90 per cent of those surveyed (including RGN, EN and degree courses) included bereavement as one of the topics taught. This was considered by the schools of nursing to have reduced anxiety in nurses dealing with death – both dying patients and bereaved relatives. However, the researchers were somewhat sceptical about the application of this to the ward situation where constraints, such as pressure of work, may prevent the objectives of the schools of nursing being put into practice. This, of course, is not unknown in other spheres of nurse education!

We exist, as nurses, to cure, or at least, to make people feel better. When we are frustrated in this aim we may react with a variety of defences such as denial, distancing, displacement and projection of negative feelings on to others. We are often close to our patients and gain much satisfaction from this. We mourn their deaths but can we cry for everyone? Can we adjust to the loss of many people we have come to like and respect?

THE BEREAVED NURSE

When we, who take on the role of nurse, are ourselves bereaved, we may find that, in order to meet the expectations of other members of our family, we are unable to grieve when we need to. We are seen as being strong or in control, and of always facing up to death and its implications. We may support and provide practical help to others, perhaps resenting a feeling of being always 'on duty'.

Crawley (1984) who founded CHAT (The Royal College of Nursing Counselling Service) found that many nurses suffered grief reactions that might, at first, appear unrelated to the original loss. This was often because they had been delayed until other family members no longer needed the nurse's support.

Who cares for the carers? is a question that is more frequently asked than in the past. A change of attitude and the provision of the resource of a trained counsellor available to everyone who works in the health services is much needed. Acknowledgement that all carers have needs as individuals has to be made by the professional as a whole. Support is *not* automatically available and has to be sought out, planned and worked at. It is *not* an optional extra but is needed by us all in whatever area we work.

Whether death is sudden or anticipated, whether it takes place in hospital or at home, it is nearly always the nurse who provides the final care to the patient and supports those most deeply affected by the loss. It is her skills of supporting, counselling, advising, educating and encouraging that are so valuable to the bereaved family.

The purpose of this book has been to provide a knowledge base on which these skills can be built. The care of the relatives is seen to be an integral part of total patient care both before and after the death of the patient.

To try to help bereaved people may seem a daunting task. The ultimate goal is well summed up by Mathers (1976), 'The pain of bereavement is the price we have to pay for loving; so that, though it is costly, it is not too dear, since the experience of losing what you have loved and grieving over it, is a challenge, to learn more about yourself, to become more mature, more healthy and truly human.'

It we can go any way towards assisting an individual to realize these goals, then a consideration of the possible needs of grieving relatives in hospital and in the community is surely both worthwhile and necessary.

REFERENCES

Birch, J. A. (1983) Anxiety and conflict in nurse education, in Davis, B. D. (ed.) *Research in Nurse Education*, Croom Helm, London.

Bloom, B. S. (1956) *Taxonomy of Educational Objectives, Handbook I: The Cognitive Domain.* Longmans Green, London.

Bowlby, J. (1981) *Attachment and Loss*, Volume 3, Penguin Books, Harmondsworth.

The Briggs Committee on Nursing (1972) *Report*, HMSO, London.

Bruner, J. S. (1966) *Towards a Theory of Instruction*, Harvard University Press, Cambridge, Mass.

Burnard, Philip (1985) *Learning Human Skills: A Guide for Nurses*, Heinemann, London.

Caughill, R. E. (1976) *The Dying Patient: A Supportive Approach*, Little, Brown and Co., Boston.

Crawley, Penny (1984) Coping with the death of a close relative. *Nursing Standard*, 25 October.

Faulkner, A. (1980) Communication and the nurse. *Nursing Times Occasional Papers*, Vol. 76 (21), pp. 93-5.

Field, D. (1984) Formal teaching in UK nursing schools about death and dying. *Medical Education*, Vol. 18, pp. 429-34.

Field, D. and Kitson, C. (1986) The practical reality. *Nursing Times*, Vol. 33 (34), 19 March.

Hopson, B. and Scally, M. (1979) *Lifeskills Teaching*, McGraw-Hill, Maidenhead.

Illich, Ivan (1976) *Limits to Medicine. Medical Nemeses: The Expropriation of Health*, Penguin Books, Harmondsworth.

Krathwohl, D. R. *et al.* (1964) *Taxonomy of Educational Objectives. Handbook 2: The Effective Domain*, David McKay, New York.

Le Shan, L. (1976) *Learning to Say Goodbye*, Macmillan, London.

Macleod Clark, J. (1981) Communication in nursing. *Nursing Times*, Vol. 77 (1), pp. 12-18.

Mathers, J. (1976) A healthy society? Reprinted in Sutherland, Ian (ed.) (1979) *Health Education: Prospectives and Choices*, Allen and Unwin Ltd., London.

Parkes, C. M. (1972) *Bereavement: Studies of Grief in Adult Life*, Tavistock, London.

Tschudin, V. (1985) Warding off a crisis. *Nursing Times*, Vol. 81(38), pp. 45-6.

Tyler, R. W. (1949) *Basic Principles of Curriculum and Instruction*, University of Chicago Press, Chicago.

Webster, M. (1981) Communicating with dying patients. *Nursing Times*, 4 June.

Worden, W. J. (1984) *Grief Counselling and Grief Therapy*, Tavistock, London.

Appendices

USEFUL ADDRESSES

Action for Victims of Medical Accident

24 Southick Street
London SE1 1TY
Tel: 081 29 12793

Age Concern

60 Pitcairn Road
Mitcham
Surrey CR4 3LL

Cruse

Cruse House
126 Sheen Road
Richmond
Surrey TW9 1UR
Tel: 081 940 4818

The Foundation for the Study of Infant Deaths
(cot death research and support)

35 Belgrave Square
London SW1X 8QB
Tel: 071 235 1721

Gingerbread

35 Wellington Street
London WC2E 7BN
Tel: 071 240 0953

Miscarriage Association

PO Box 24
Osset
West Yorks WF5 9XG
Tel: 0924 830515

The National Society for the Mentally Handicapped

117–123 Golden Lane
London EC17 ORT

Parents of Murdered Children Support Group
(part of Compassionate Friends)

c/o 10 Eastern Avenue
Prittlewell
Southend
Essex SS2 5QU
Tel: 0702 68510

Patients Association

Room 33
18 Charing Cross Road
London WC2H 0HR
Tel: 071 240 0671

PETS (Pre-eclamptic Toxaemia Society)

Dawn James, Ty Iago
High Street
Llanbers
Gwynedd LL5B 4HB
Tel: 0286 872477

SAFTA (support after termination for fetal abnormality)

29–30 Soho Square
London W1V 6JB
Tel: 071 439 6124

SANDS (Stillbirth and Neonatal Death Society)

28 Portland Place
London W1 4DE
Tel: 071 436 5881

Society of Compassionate Friends (parents who have lost a child)

6 Denmark Street
Bristol BS1 5DQ
Tel: 0272 292778

Terrence Higgins Trust (Aids patients and their families)

52-54 Grays Inn Road
London WC1X 8JU
Tel: 071 831 0330

FURTHER READING

Age Concern, *Bereavement and the Elderly: A Training Aid*, Age Concern, Mitcham.

Bowlby, J. *Attachment and Loss*, Vol. 1: *Attachment* (1969) Vol. 2: *Separation* (1973), Vol. 3: *Loss* (1980) Hogarth Press, London.

Charles-Edwards, A. (1983) *The Nursing Care of the Dying Patient*, Beaconsfield Publishers Ltd, Beaconsfield.

Frankl, Victor (1963) *Man's Search for Meaning*, Beacon Press, London.

Freud, S. (1917) *Mourning and Melancholia*, Hogarth Press, London (1957).

Fulton, R. (1977) *Death Grief and Bereavement, A Bibliography 1945–1975*, Arno Press, New York.

Gorer, G. (1965) *Death, Grief and Mourning in Contemporary Britain*, Cresset Press, London.

Hill, Susan (1986) *In the Springtime of the Year*, Penguin, Harmondsworth.

Hinton, John (1974) *Dying*, Penguin, Harmondsworth.

Hopson, B. and Scally M. (1978) *Lifeskills Teaching*, McGraw-Hill, Maidenhead.

Kalish, R. A. (1977) *Death and Dying, Views from Many Cultures*, Baywood Inc., New Jersey.

Kennedy, Eugene (1983) *On Becoming a Counsellor: A Basic Guide for Non-professional Counsellors*, Gill and Macmillan Ltd, Dublin.

Kubler-Ross, E. (1970) *On Death and Dying*, Tavistock, London.

Kubler-Ross, E. (1984) *Questions and Answers on Death and Dying*, Macmillan, London.

Lake, Tony (1984) *Living with Grief*, Sheldon Press, London.

Marris, Peter (1986) *Loss and Change*, Routledge and Kegan Paul, London.

Neuberger, Julia (1987) *Caring for Dying People of Different Faiths*, The Lisa Sainsbury Foundation, Croydon.

Parkes, C. M. (1972) *Bereavement: Studies of Grief in Adult Life*, Tavistock, London.

Parkes, C. M. and Weiss, R. S. (1983) *Recovery from Bereavement*, Basic Books, Inc., New York.

Raphael, Beverly (1985) *The Anatomy of Bereavement*, Hutchinson, London.

Robbins, Joy (1989) *Caring for the Dying Patient and the Family* (Lippincott Nursing Series), Harper and Row, London.

Ryan, C. and Ryan, K. (1980) *A Private Battle*, New English Library, London.

Schiff, Harriet (1979) *The Bereaved Parent*, Souvenir Press, London.

Sheey, G. (1977) *Passages: Predictable Crises of Adult Life*, Dutton, New York.

Speck, Peter (1978) *Loss and Grief in Medicine*, Baillière Tindall, London.

Stedeford, Averil (1984) *Facing Death*, Heinemann, London.

Stoebe, W. and Stoebe, M. S. (1987) *Bereavement and Health*, Cambridge University Press, Cambridge.

Viost, Judith (1986) *Necessary Losses*, Simon and Schuster, New York.

Ward, Barbara and Houghton, Jamie (1987) *Good Grief – Talking and Learning about Loss and Death* (teaching pack), Cruse Publications, London.

Wright, Bob (1986) *Caring in Crisis: A Handbook of Intervention Skills for Nurses*, Churchill Livingstone, London.

RESOURCES

The Lisa Sainsbury Foundation, 8–10 Crown Hill, Croydon, Surrey, CR0 1RY (Tel: 081 686 8808) hold a very useful library of videos and tapes and can provide book reviews on death and bereavement.

The Information Centre, St Christopher's Hospice, Sydenham, London (Tel: 081 778 9252) has a library of books and audiovisual materials, and provides information on all aspects of cancer care, death and bereavement.

Index

Abortion 74
  after amniocentesis 75–76
Acceptance, in adjustment 37–38
Adjustment, stages of 35–39
  acceptance 37–38
  anger, rage, resentment 36
  bargaining 37
  denial 35–36
  depression 37
Adolescents, bereavement in 84–90
  concept of death 84–85
  mourning process in 87
  parents' death 85–86
  pseudoadult behaviour in 89
Adulthood, death in 92–109
Advice, giving 127
Aesthetic needs 116
Afterlife, belief in 22
Agoraphobia, study 65
Aids 104–107
  bisexuals 106
  Buddy system of help 106
  and drug addicts 107
  HIV infection 104
  homosexuals 105
  Terrence Higgins Trust 106
Aimlessness, as bereavement process 7–8
Ambivalent relationships, at risk group 67
Amniocentesis, and abortion 75–76
Amputation, loss after 3
Anger
  in adjustment 36
  in bereavement process 6–7

  at God 7
Anniversaries, vulnerability of 142
Anticipated death 47–48
Apathy, as bereavement process 7–8
At risk groups 66–69, 73–91, 92, 109
  ambivalent relationships 67
  children and adolescents 84–90
  in death by disaster 103–107
  in death by violence 100–103
  image-conscious individual 66–67
  isolated individuals 67–68
  losing a child before or after birth 73–84
  mental handicap 108
  old age 96–100
  overdependent relationships 68–69
  past history of emotional crisis 69
  suicide 92–96
Awareness context 35

Baby
  funeral service for 78
  keepsakes and memories 77
  naming 77
Bakongo tribe, Zaire 19
Bargaining, in adjustment 37
Basic needs 111–114
  aesthetic 116
  cognitive 116
  to cope with vulnerable times 112
  love and belonging 115
  for others 113
  for physical health and fitness 111–112
  safety 115

security 111
self-esteem 115
for self-indulgence 114
stability 112–113
Bereaved
    elderly parents 97–100
    nurse 163–164
    visiting 147–150
Bereavement
    aims of help in 125–126
    in children and adolescents 84–90
        concept of death 84–85
    counselling service 95, 108, 128, 145–147, 161
    defining 1–15
    elderly parents 97–100
    factors affecting outcome 64
    and Grief, International Conference 86
    practical help 132–133
    as a process 4–5
        disengagement, apathy, aimlessness 7–8
        hope and new directions 8–9
        shock, numbness and pain of grieving 4–5
        showing fear, guilt and anger, and resentment 5–7
        time scale 63
    'quiz' 137
    as a series of tasks 9–10
        accepting reality of loss 9, 12
        adjusting to a new environment 9–10
    experiencing pain and grief 9
    withdrawing emotional energy and reinvesting in other relationships 10
    statements 136–143
    support, services involved 120, 123
        planning 123–125
    as a transition 10–13
        depression 12
        immobilization 11–12
        internalization 13
        meaning, searching for 13
        minimization 12
        testing 12
    visits, guidelines for helpers 143–145
        observation, practical problems 144
Biological death 46–47
Bisexuals and Aids 106
Bloom's categories of cognitive domain 156
Body, seeing 57–58
Bradford football disaster 103
Brain death 104
Breastfeeding, and sudden infant death syndrome 81
Briggs Committee on Nursing 161
Buddy help system, in Aids 106
Buffalo Creek disaster 103

Burial 20
Burn out 152, 162

Cancer 5, 37, 74, 105
    National Society for Relief 47
Carcinoma, of lung 32, 38
Care
    in the community 118–134
    involvement in 33–34
    primary health team 120–123
Case studies, in education and training 158
CHAT (Royal College of Nursing Counselling Service) 164
Child
    death of 83
    losing before or after birth 73–84
        abortion 74–76
        infertility 73
        miscarriage 74
        stillbirth 76–78
    regression in 86
Children
    bereavement in 84–90
        attendance at funeral 90
        Northern Ireland study 85
        parents' death 85–86
    and death 73–91
    and divorce 2
Chorion villus sampling 76
Clergy 52–53
Cognitive needs 116
Colostomy nurse 43
Communication, skills 136–152
    bereavement 'quiz' 137
    techniques 151
Community
    care in 118–134
        information, links with hospital 119
        services 121
    nurse 41
Compassion fatigue 162
Coronary artery disease 123
Coroner, duty in sudden infant death syndrome 80
Cot death (see Sudden infant death sydrome)
Counselling service, bereavement 95, 108, 128, 145–147, 161
    Royal College of Nursing (CHAT) 164
    Wessex model 145–146
Cruse (Association for Widows and Widowers) 68, 95, 130, 166
Cryopreservation 22
Cremation 19, 20, 21
Culture, customs and rituals 16–26

Death
  in adulthood 92–109
  anticipated 47–48
  biological 46–47
  brain 104
  of child 83
  and children 73–91
  to be done at 55
  family needs after 110–117
  in intensive care 104
  neonatal 78–79
  Oxford Book 17
  of parent 85–86
  'pornography' of 17
  psychological 46
  of sibling 87
  social 46
  sudden 69–71
  sudden infant, syndrome 80–82
  time of 59–60
  unexpected infant 79–80
Denial, in adjustment 35–36
Department of Social Security 121
Depression 8, 12, 65
  in adjustment 37
Diaries, as therapy 132
Direct action 128
Disaster, death from 103
  Bradford, Buffalo Creek,
    Hillsborough 103
Disengagement, as bereavement process 7–8
District nursing sister 120–121
Divorce 2–4
  and children 2
Drug addicts, and Aids 107
Dying patient 42
Dying trajectory 35

Education and training 156–161
  case studies 158
  formal lectures 158
  reinforcement 159
  role-play 159
  workshops 159
Elderly parents, bereaved 97–100
Emotional crisis, past history 69
Energy, emotional, withdrawing 10
Environment, adjusting to new 9–10
Evaluation 126–127
  outcome and process 126

Falklands war (1982) 70
Family needs
  after the patient's death 110–117
  before the patient's death 27–43
  at the patient's death 45–60

Fear, in bereavement process 5, 40
Foundation for the Study of Infant
    Deaths 81, 167
Frankl, Victor 13
Freud, concept of grief-work 9, 10
Funeral 18, 19–25
  after 54
  attendance of children at 90
  arranging 56
  director 53–56
  function of 23–25
  role of in mourning 23

God, anger at 7
Grief,
  and Bereavement, International
    Conference 86
  'double' 71
  experiencing 9
  reactions, unresolved 65–66, 81
Grief-work, Freud's concept 9
Grieving
  complicated, clues to indicate 62–65
  patterns of 61
  pain of, in bereavement process 4–5
Guilt
  in bereavement process 5–6
    and mourning 6
  feelings of 149

Health visitor 43, 121
Help
  aims in bereavement 125–126
  Buddy system, in Aids 106
  communication skills 136–152
  media 132
  practical 132–133
  tools for 150–151
Helping strategies 127–129
  counselling 129
  direct action 128
  giving advice 127
  giving information 127–128
  system change 128–129
  teaching 128
Helplessness, feelings of 36
Hillsborough disaster 103
HIV infection 104, 106
Holmes and Rahe readjustment scales 13,
    14
Home care
  Macmillan services 134
  versus hospital care 33
Homosexuals and Aids 105
Hope
  in bereavement process 8–9
  relatives' need for 31–32

Hospice 120
  movement 47
  nurses 54
  St Christopher's, Sydenham 47, 95
Hospital care
  links with community 119
  versus home care 33
Hungerford massacre 102

Image-conscious individual, at risk 66–67
Immobilization 11–12
Infant death
  Foundation for Study 81, 167
  sudden, syndrome (SIDS) 80–82
  unexpected 79–80
Infertility 73
Information
  giving 127–128
  need for 29–30
Inquest, in death by violence 83–84
Intensive care, deaths in 104
Internalization 13
Isolated individuals, at risk 67–68
Israel, wars in 101

Jews 24
  and death by violence 101

Kalil Gibran 45
Kohner Report on Midwives and Stillbirths
  (1984) 76
Kubler-Ross, E. 35, 38, 39

Lectures, in education and training 158
Liaison sister 43, 122–123
Libraries 132
A Little Lifetime 77–78
Loss
  accepting reality of 9
  amputation 3–9
  as a key concept 2
  in old age 96–97
  of a pet 2
  of a precious object 3
  and terminal illness 6
  through violence 100–103
Love
  and belonging need 115
  'remembering with' 98–100

Macmillan Unit 120
  family evenings 131
  Christchurch 30, 47
  home care services 134
  nurses 54
Maslow's hierarchy of needs 114, 116
Meaning, search for 13

Media help 132
Memorials 20, 21
Mental handicap 108
Midwives 122
  Kohner Report 76
Minimization 12
Miscarriage 74
Moslems 24
Mourning
  and guilt 6
  process in adolescents 87
  prolonged or complicated 61–72
  role of funeral in 23
Myocardial infarction 70, 71

National Society for Cancer Relief 47
Needs
  after the death 110–117
    identifying basic 111–114
    Maslow's hierarchy 114
    physiological 114–115
  family, before patient's death 27–43
    information 29–30
    involvement in care 33–34
    hope 31–32
    home or hospital 33
    relatives 28–29
    telling the truth 39–43
    timescale of illness 34–39
    visiting times 30–31
  family at patient's death 45–60
    social, psychological, biological
      death 46–47
  patient's 48–53
  relatives' emotional 50
Neonatal death 78–79
  SANDS (Stillbirth and Neonatal Death
    Society) 77, 168
New directions, and bereavement
  process 8–9
Next of kin 3
Northern Ireland, study of children in 85
Numbness, in bereavement process 4–5
Nurse
  bereaved 163–164
  colostomy 43
  community 41
  hospice 54
  liaison 122
  practice 122
  selection, support and education
    for 154–164
  specialist 122
Nursing
  Briggs Committee on 161
  Royal College Counselling Service
    (CHAT) 164

schools, studies 162

Occupational health departments 161
Old age, loss in 96-97
Overdependent relationships, at risk 68-69
Oxford Book of Death 17

Paediatrician, interview with 81
Pain, experiencing 9
Parents
  bereaved elderly 97-100
  death of 85-86
Patient
  death, family needs before 27-43
  dying 42
  needs 48-53
    physical 48-52
    psychological 50-51
    social 51-52
    spiritual 52-53
Phobias 65
Physical needs 48-50
  health and fitness 111-112
Physiological needs 114-115
Physiotherapist 43
Pilgrim Club 131
Planning, in bereavement support 123-125
  potential problems 124-125
Post-mortems 25
  in death by violence 83
  in sudden infant death syndrome 80
Practical help, in bereavement 132-133,
  139, 140
  diaries 132-133
  libraries 132
  from the media 132
Practice nurses 122
Pregnancy 75
Primary health care team 120-123
  district nursing sister 120-121
  health visitor 43, 121
  practice nurses 122
Pseudoadult behaviour, in adolescents 89
Psychological death 46
Psychological needs 50-51

Queen Victoria, and Prince Albert 66

Rage, in adjustment 36
Readjustment scales, Holmes and Rahe 13,
  14
Reality, acceptance 12
Reinforcement 159
Relate (marriage guidance) 129
Relationships
  new 10
  overdependent, at risk 68-69

Relatives' needs, before patient's
  death 28-29
  information 29-30
Relaxation techniques 149
Remembrance, garden 21
Resentment
  in adjustment 36
  in bereavement process 5-7
Ritual, culture and customs 16-26
Role-play, in education and training 159
Royal College of Nursing Counselling
  Service (CHAT) 164

Safety needs 115
Samaritans 129
SANDS (Stillbirth and Neonatal Death
  Society) 77, 168
Security needs 111
Selective forgetting 35
Self-actualization 116-117
Self-esteem 115
Self-help groups 129-131
  Cruse 68, 95, 130, 166
  informal 131
Self-indulgence, need for 114
Sen, Amartya 86
Shock, in bereavement process 4-5
  shell 11
Shrine, creating 62
Siblings
  death of 87
  and sudden infant death syndrome 81
Sir Michael Sobell House, Oxford 133
Sleep, inducing 81, 140
Social circle, exclusion from 141
Social death 46
Social isolation 95
Social needs 51-52
Social services 121
Spiritual needs 52-53
Stability needs 112-113
Staff selection 155-163
  education and training 156-161
    Bloom's categories of cognitive
      domain 156
St Christopher's Hospice, Syndenham 47
  bereavement counselling service 95
  Pilgrim Club 131
Stillbirth 76-78
  Kohner Report 76
Sudden infant death syndrome (SIDS) 80-82
  checklist for 80
Suicide 92-96
  fear 93
Support groups 162-163
Sympathy, giving 139

Teaching
  as a helping strategy 127–129
  Tyler's model 159–160
Terminal illness 6
Terrence Higgins Trust 106, 168
Tibetan Book of the Dead 18
Timescale, of illness 34–35
Transition process 10–13
  immobilization 11–12
  model 11
Truth, to tell or not 39–43
  and charity 41
  Russian study 41
Tyler's model of teaching and
    learning 159–160

Useful addresses 166–168

Violence, death by 83–84, 100–103
Visiting the bereaved 147–150
Visiting times 30–31
Volunteer schemes 133–134

Wakes 22, 23
Wessex Model of Counselling 145–146
Widows
  Cruse (Association for) 68, 95, 130, 166
  study of London 94
Workshops, in education and training 159

Zaire, Bakongo tribe 19